AF715147

Table of Con[illegible]

KETO POWER
BY
LENIN DEV

Copyright

Published by: Phoenix Wings Press LLC

Email: phoenixwingspress@gmail.com

First Edition

Disclaimer

This book is intended for informational and educational purposes only and is not intended as medical advice. The content provided is based on the author's personal research, experience, and interpretation of available knowledge at the time of writing.

Always consult with your physician, dietitian, or other qualified healthcare provider before beginning any new dietary or lifestyle program. Individual results may vary, and no guarantees are made regarding specific outcomes. The author and publisher disclaim all liability for any loss or injury caused directly or indirectly by the information in this book.

About the Author

Lenin Dev is a passionate wellness writer and lifestyle strategist who specializes in helping people reclaim their health through simple, sustainable changes. With a deep interest in nutritional science, fitness, and mindset, Lenin empowers readers to take charge of their bodies, break free from fad diets, and achieve lasting transformation.

When not writing Lenin enjoys nature walks, strong coffee, and inspiring others to live with purpose, energy, and intention.

Acknowledgments

To the incredible individuals who've shared their keto success stories — your journeys were a source of inspiration throughout the writing of this book.

To my readers — thank you for trusting me as your guide. It is your dedication to health and growth that keeps this mission alive.

And finally, to anyone taking the first step toward transformation — remember, the power is already within you. Keep going.

CHAPTER 1 — INTRODUCTION TO KETO POWER

The ketogenic lifestyle is a remarkable path forward for anyone who wants to transform their health, their energy, their body, and their mind. It's a way of living that finds its roots in the very physiology of human metabolism, a powerful approach to nourishment that reshapes the way we produce and use energy on a daily basis. At its core, the ketogenic diet focuses on a dramatic reduction in carbohydrate intake while emphasizing healthy fats and a proper amount of proteins. It's a metabolic shift — a deep, profound change — in the way your body converts food into energy and performs its countless daily operations.

When you first embark on a ketogenic journey, you are making a dramatic break from the diet that most people follow today — a diet heavy in processed carbohydrates, added sugars, and a constant stream of glucose. Naturally, your body has become conditioned over years or decades to rely predominantly on glucose — a simple form of sugar — for its primary energy. Your muscles, your brain, and your cells have gotten used to a constant delivery of carbohydrate-fueled energy, and this dependence has a dramatic ripple effect on your health, your metabolic flexibility, and your ability to manage hunger and energy levels. The ketogenic diet converts this process from a sugar-centric view to a state where your body efficiently produces energy from fats and ketones.

Ketones are small, powerful molecules that your liver produces when carbohydrate intake drops and your body starts breaking down fatty acids for energy. Instead of running on glucose — a less efficient and more reactive form of energy — your body converts fatty acids into ketone bodies — predominantly beta-hydroxybutyrate, acetoacetate, and acetone — which become a stable, abundant, and clean-burning energy for both your body and your mind. There's a remarkable transformation when your body starts to use ketones predominantly; many people report sustained energy without the dramatic drops and cravings that typically come after consuming a carbohydrate-rich meal.

This shift toward a ketogenic state brings numerous health benefits that have made this lifestyle profoundly popular across health, fitness, and wellness communities. The first and most immediately noticeable benefit for many is weight loss. Naturally, when your body starts to use its own stores of fatty acids for energy instead of constantly depending on a stream of incoming carbohydrates, it begins to break down its own body fat. That means you're not just cutting calories; you're turning your body into a literal "fat-burning machine." Importantly, this process occurs without the dramatic drops in energy and persistent hunger signals that typically undermine restrictive dieting. Your body finds a deep, sustained energy from its own stores and from the healthy fats you consume.

But the benefits of a ketogenic lifestyle go far beyond simply dropping excess weight. The diet has powerful effects on metabolic health, improving insulin resistance, reducing the risk of Type 2 diabetes, and helping stabilize blood sugar. Furthermore, many people find their cravings diminish profoundly once their body enters a state of ketosis. Without the rollercoaster of glucose and insulin, the signals for hunger become more reliable, more appropriate to their true energy needs. Instead of feeling constantly driven by a need to eat, people find peace and control in their food choices. They learn to appreciate true, deep satiety and become less obsessed with their next meal.

This newfound stability extends to energy and mental clarity. Your brain, which normally relies on glucose for its main energy, finds a rich, uninterrupted stream of energy in ketones. The result is often described as a dramatic reduction in "fog"— a clearer, more focused mind. Your ability to concentrate, solve problems, and perform mental tasks improves. Furthermore, many people report a more stable mood and less irritability once their body converts to this alternative energy state. Without the dramatic fluctuations in blood sugar, you become less prone to the dramatic drops in energy and mood that often follow a carbohydrate-rich meal. Instead, you enjoy a sustained, clear, and calm mental state.

Physical performance can be profoundly influenced by this change in energy utilization. Although there may be a brief period of adaptation — sometimes called the "keto flu"— during which your body adjusts its metabolic machinery, many people find their physical endurance and recovery improve once they become proficient at burning fats for energy.

Distance runners, for example, appreciate having nearly unlimited energy from their own body's fat stores, instead of needing to constantly refuel with carbohydrate gels and drinks. Naturally, this makes the ketogenic lifestyle particularly useful for sustained, low-intensity physical activity and for people who wish to avoid dramatic fluctuations in their energy and performance.

As you progress further into a ketogenic lifestyle, your body adapts at a deep, cellular level. The metabolic pathways that produce ketones become more efficient; the number and size of mitochondria — your cells' power stations — increase; and you become proficient at accessing and utilizing fatty acids for energy. The result is a dramatic improvement in metabolic health and flexibility. Your body is no longer a fragile system that depends on a constant infusion of carbohydrate; instead, it finds its energy within its own stores and from a diet rich in healthy fats and proteins.

This process profoundly impacts health markers across numerous dimensions. People following a ketogenic diet often find their cholesterol profile improving, their HDL (the "good" cholesterol) increasing, and their triglycerides dropping. Furthermore, their blood pressure may stabilize, and markers of chronic inflammation diminish. There's growing research suggesting that this lifestyle may be protective against a range of health conditions — from Type 2 diabetes and obesity to neurodegenerative disorders and even certain forms of cancer — by reducing oxidative stress, improving mitochondrial health, and dampening chronic inflammation.

Because this approach brings about a fundamental shift in the way your body produces energy and signals satiety, it naturally guides you toward consuming a diet rich in whole, unprocessed foods. Foods like avocado, fatty fish, grass-fed meats, olive oil, and low-carbohydrate vegetables become your staples. The result is a dramatic reduction in processed food, added sugars, and refined carbohydrates — a change that further supports health and well-being.

This diet is not a temporary fix. It's a powerful, sustainable way of living — a lifestyle — that brings a deep and lasting transformation. Your body evolves into a proficient fat-burner, a state you can maintain for years to come. The result is a remarkable combination of health, energy, and peace — a deep, clear, sustained vitality that lets you pursue your goals and passions without being held back by fluctuations in energy or health.

Your ability to stay in this state depends not on willpower or restrictive calorie counting but on honoring your body's true physiology. It involves choosing foods that align with your metabolic needs and letting your body do what it was designed to do — efficiently produce energy from its own resources.

This is the power of the ketogenic lifestyle. It transforms not just your physical health but your mental clarity, your energy, and your ability to live a rich, engaged, and active life. It's a powerful tool for unlocking your body's potential — a potential that lies within each of us — to become the fullest, healthiest, most energetic version of ourselves. It's a way of honoring our physiology, aligning our diet with our biology, and experiencing health from the inside out.

As you progress further into this lifestyle, you become more and more proficient at choosing foods that align with this metabolic state. Your grocery list evolves; it starts to reflect a rich array of whole, unprocessed ingredients — fatty cuts of grass-fed meats, wild-caught fish rich in omega-3s, a spectrum of colorful, low-carbohydrate vegetables, avocado, olives, and a range of healthy fats from sources like coconut oil and ghee. Naturally, you move away from processed products, from the typical ultra-processed foods that were designed in a laboratory to appeal to your taste buds and undermine your ability to regulate your own appetite.

This process not only transforms your physical health; it also reconnects you with the rich, pleasurable experience of food in its pure form. Your senses become more acute; your taste buds start to appreciate the subtleties in a piece of grilled wild-caught salmon or a perfectly ripened avocado. The rich texture of a fatty cut of steak or the creamy softness of a pastured-egg omelette become sources of deep satisfaction, a dramatic shift from the momentary, fleeting rush you previously experienced from a piece of candy or a bag of chips.

This newfound satisfaction plays a key role in reducing cravings and binge-like behaviors. Naturally, when you nourish your body with foods rich in healthy fats, proteins, and fiber, you activate signals of satiety and well-being. Your body responds by dialing back its signals to constantly search for more food. It's a powerful reversal of the chronic hunger signals that many people suffer from when their diet consists predominantly of processed carbohydrates and sugars.

Your pancreas, which previously kept sending signals to release large amounts of insulin to deal with excess glucose, starts to normalize its activity. Your cells become more sensitive to insulin; you find yourself needing less and less of it to regulate your blood sugar. The result is less stress on your pancreas, lower baseline insulin levels, and a dramatic reduction in your risk of developing Type 2 diabetes and metabolic syndrome.

Your liver, a key metabolic organ, also finds renewal in this process. Instead of constantly converting excess glucose into fatty deposits — a phenomenon called fatty liver — it starts to clear those deposits and heal. Naturally, this can lead to a resolution of non-alcoholic fatty liver disease, a condition that has become alarmingly prevalent in modern society and is a key driver of metabolic dysfunction.

Meanwhile, your muscles become proficient at using fatty acids and ketones for energy, and your mitochondria — the tiny powerhouses within your cells — become more numerous and more efficient. The result is a dramatic improvement in physical and mental energy, a newfound ability to perform daily tasks, pursue physical goals, and appreciate life without the persistent feeling of weakness or lethargy.

This transformation occurs not just at the macronutrient level — shifting from carbohydrates to fats — but at the most fundamental level of your physiology. Your body is designed to be flexible, adaptable, and proficient at using whatever sources of energy are available. The ketogenic diet simply reconnects you with this ability — a ability that your ancestors relied upon for millennia in an environment where food was not always abundant and carbohydrates were scarce. Naturally, this makes you more resilient and less prone to fluctuations in energy, mood, and health.

This adaptability has a dramatic ripple effect on numerous aspects of health. Your cardiovascular health, for example, starts to improve. Lowering carbohydrate intake reduces the production of small, dense LDL particles — the form of LDL most strongly associated with atherosclerosis — while boosting HDL, the protective form of cholesterol. Furthermore, your triglycerides drop and your ratio of HDL to triglycerides — a powerful indicator of metabolic health — improves.

Your blood pressure may normalize as well, reflecting a reduction in chronic inflammation, a drop in sodium retention, and an improvement in arterial stiffness. The result is a lowered risk of developing heart disease and stroke — two leading causes of death in the modern world.

Meanwhile, your body's ability to regulate inflammation at the cellular level is profoundly influenced by this metabolic shift. The production of reactive oxygen species drops, and the activity of powerful antioxidant systems within your cells — such as glutathione — increases. The result is a dramatic reduction in chronic, low-grade inflammation — a key driver of numerous diseases of lifestyle.

Your gut, a rich ecosystem of microorganisms, responds positively as well. The ketogenic diet typically reduces the intake of processed carbohydrates and added sugars — two components that can foster an imbalance in gut flora and promote the growth of harmful microbial species. Instead, by emphasizing whole, natural foods rich in fiber and healthy fats, you foster a more balanced and diverse microbial community — a community that produces compounds protective against disease and supportive of a strong immune system.

Your mental health, meanwhile, may find renewal in this lifestyle. The ketogenic diet has a rich history of use in epilepsy, particularly for children with medication-resistant seizures. Today, research is exploring its potential benefits for conditions ranging from Alzheimer's and Parkinson's to autism, bipolar disorder, and depression. The mechanisms are not yet fully understood, but it's clear that shifting the brain's main energy from glucose to ketones profoundly influences neuronal stability, neuroinflammation, and neurodegenerative processes.

Some people find that their memory, mood, and ability to concentrate all improve on a ketogenic diet. There's a growing body of research suggesting that ketones act not just as a metabolic substrate — a form of energy — but also as signaling molecules, influencing the expression of genes related to stress resistance, neuroplasticity, and neuronal health. Furthermore, a ketogenic diet may help to regulate the production of neurochemicals, reducing glutamate — an excitatory transmitter — and strengthening GABA — a calming transmitter — thereby contributing to a more stable and resilient nervous system.

CHAPTER 2 — WHY KETO WORKS

From the moment you embark on a ketogenic lifestyle, you realize something profoundly different is happening within you. The path you're choosing isn't just another diet — it's a dramatic, powerful metabolic transformation. It's a renewal at the most fundamental level of physiology, a shift that lets your body break free from the restrictive view that all diet success comes down to counting calories and suffering through persistent hunger and cravings. Instead, a ketogenic diet guides you back toward a more natural way of fueling your body — a way that lets you become a proficient, flexible, and efficient fat-burner.

For years, many people were told that weight control was a simple matter of "calories in and calories out." If you burned more calories than you consumed, you'd lose weight; if you ate more than you burned, you'd gain it. But this view disregards a key piece of human physiology: not all calories affect your body in the same way. The macronutrient composition of your diet — whether it's predominantly carbohydrate, protein, or fat — profoundly influences your hormonal signals, your metabolic pathways, and your ability to tap into your own body's stored energy.

This is where ketogenic dieting diverges from the calorie-centric view. Traditionally, many diet plans rely on a reduced calorie intake while still emphasizing carbohydrates as a main energy source. The result is a temporary drop in weight — mainly water and muscle — but it's a drop that often comes with persistent hunger, cravings, and eventual plateaus. Your body resists this form of weight loss by slowing its metabolic rate and conserving energy. It's a survival mechanism hard-wired into you from an ancestral past when food scarcity was a constant pressure. Furthermore, a calorie-restricted, carbohydrate-rich diet makes you more prone to fluctuations in blood sugar and insulin, adding to the feeling of weakness and persistent hunger.

Ketogenic dieting, in contrast, cuts carbohydrate intake profoundly, typically to less than 50 grams per day — sometimes even lower. That dramatic reduction signals your body to enter a state called ketosis. Instead of depending on glucose — a form of sugar — for its primary energy, your body starts to break down fatty acids into small molecules called ketones. These ketones become a powerful and clean energy source for your muscles, your brain, and your other tissues. Naturally, this reduces your reliance on a constant supply of carbohydrates and lets you tap into the vast stores of energy already within you — your own body fat.

This process transforms your metabolic physiology in numerous ways. First and foremost, it lets you lose excess body-fat faster and more sustained over time, without the muscle wasting that often occurs in calorie-restricted dieting. Traditionally, when you cut calories, your body may break down muscle in addition to fat, adding to weakness and slowing your metabolic rate. But in a state of ketosis, muscle is largely preserved; your body has a rich, abundant supply of energy from its own fatty deposits, which spares muscle from being catabolized.

Meanwhile, your hunger signals diminish. Naturally, a diet rich in healthy fats and proteins is more satiating and more slowly digested, and the production of ketones itself seems to dampen the signals of hunger in your brain. Furthermore, without dramatic fluctuations in blood sugar and insulin — fluctuations that typically follow a carbohydrate-rich meal — your body finds it easier to regulate its own appetite. It signals when you're adequately fueled and dampens those persistent cravings for more food. Eating transforms from a compulsion into a conscious, purposeful act — a dramatic change in your relationship with food.

This reduction in hunger signals makes a ketogenic diet much more sustainable over the long term. Instead of battling your physiology, you align with it. Naturally, you eat less without feeling deprived. The diet's ability to stabilize blood sugar and diminish the dramatic swings in insulin has numerous health benefits. It reduces the risk of developing Type 2 diabetes and metabolic disorders, and it can help reverse those conditions in people who already suffer from them. There is growing clinical and research evidence that a ketogenic diet profoundly improves markers of metabolic health — from reduced fasting glucose and lower Hemoglobin A1c to improved HDL and reduced triglycerides.

Furthermore, this lifestyle lets you break free from the restrictive view that all calories are equal and that weight control is simply a mathematical equation. Instead, it underscores a more sophisticated view — a view that you are a complex, adaptable biochemical system. The signals you send to your body through diet profoundly affect its physiology. Eating a diet rich in healthy fats, proteins, and low in carbohydrates signals your body to become proficient at accessing its own energy stores. It transforms you from a person who is constantly dependent on a stream of food into a person who is flexible, resilient, and proficient at using its own resources.

This view has powerful implications not just for weight control but for health in a much broader sense. Metabolic disorders — from diabetes and obesity to fatty liver and polycystic ovary syndrome — all reflect a deep dysfunction in the body's ability to regulate energy. The ketogenic diet directly addresses this dysfunction by removing the excess carbohydrate signals and allowing the body to revert to its native, healthy metabolic state.

In this context, a ketogenic diet isn't a temporary fix or a restrictive regimen — it's a powerful, sustainable way of living. It lets you align your physiology with your lifestyle and break free from the diet rollercoaster. Naturally, when your body finds its own balance, excess weight drops away, health markers improve, and energy levels stabilize. It's a transformation from the inside — a renewal at the most fundamental level — and it highlights the dramatic power of diet to affect not just your physical appearance, but your health, well-being, and future.

As you progress further into a ketogenic lifestyle, something remarkable happens: your body starts to become more proficient at accessing its own resources. The metabolic machinery within your cells — particularly within your mitochondria — upregulates the production of the enzymes required to break down fatty acids efficiently and to produce ketones in the liver. It's a form of metabolic training; just as your muscles become strong and conditioned through physical exercise, your ability to use fat for energy becomes more robust through this lifestyle. Naturally, this means you become less dependent on the next meal for energy and more proficient at drawing from your own abundant stores.

This adaptability has a dramatic ripple effect on your day-to-day energy. Without dramatic drops in blood sugar or the "crash" that typically follows a carbohydrate-rich meal, your energy becomes more stable and sustained. The result is greater physical and mental endurance — whether you're going for a run, lifting weights, or simply focusing on your work — your body and mind are fueled by a deep, rich, and reliable energy reserve.

This metabolic shift underscores another key advantage of the ketogenic diet over calorie-restricted, carbohydrate-heavy plans: it transforms your relationship to food. Naturally, when you're less driven by fluctuations in blood sugar and less prone to hunger signals, you find it easier to implement a form of intermittent fasting — simply extending the periods between your meals. This isn't a form of restrictive suffering; instead, it feels effortless, because your body isn't begging you for a constant delivery of glucose. It's proficient at accessing its own resources and converts them into energy smoothly and efficiently. This phenomenon — often called "fat-adaptation"— lets you go for extended periods without food and without experiencing weakness or hunger.

Furthermore, this ability to fast safely and comfortably brings additional health benefits. Fasting has a powerful effect on numerous metabolic pathways — it reduces insulin, drops blood sugar, and signals the body to clear damaged components through a process called autophagy. Autophagy is a kind of cellular renewal; it destroys and recycles faulty components, making way for the growth of healthy, functional ones. Naturally, this process reduces the risk of age-related disorders, from neurodegenerative conditions to cardiovascular disease and diabetes. Ketogenic dieting, by reducing reliance on glucose and reducing meal frequency, lets you activate these powerful mechanisms without stress or suffering.

Meanwhile, from a hormonal standpoint, the diet profoundly dampens the signals that promote fat storage and metabolic dysfunction. Insulin, a key storage hormone, drops, reducing the signals to store excess calories in your fat cells. At the same time, glucagon — a counterpart to insulin — increases, helping to release fatty acids from storage and mobilize them for energy. This shift in the insulin-to-glucagon ratio signals to your body that it's a time of renewal and utilization, not storage — which is precisely what you want for sustained weight control and health improvement.

Furthermore, this state has powerful effects on two key regulators of metabolism: AMP-activated protein kinase (AMPK) and mammalian target of rapamycin (mTOR). AMPK is a kind of metabolic "master switch" that signals your body to increase energy production and break down stored components when energy is scarce. Ketogenic dieting naturally stimulates AMPK, putting you into a more youthful, vigorous, and adaptive metabolic state. Meanwhile, mTOR, a growth and storage signal, drops during ketogenic dieting — reducing signals for growth and instead allowing your body to focus on maintenance, repair, and renewal. This balance — less mTOR, more AMPK — underpins many of the health and longevity benefits that come with a ketogenic lifestyle.

Your body, in this state, is not weak or starving; it's flexible, strong, and purposeful. It's a dramatic contrast to the weak, hungry feeling that typically characterises calorie-restricted dieting. Instead of conserving energy and slowing its metabolic rate, your body maintains its ability to produce energy at a high level — while drawing it from its own stores instead of from a constant stream of food.

This has a powerful psychological component as well. Because your body is well-fueled and your brain has a reliable energy supply, you find it easier to avoid impulsive decisions driven by low blood sugar and cravings. Your willpower grows stronger, not because you're forcing it, but because you're no longer battling powerful signals from your physiology. This reduces stress, makes lifestyle choices more effortless, and lets you align your behavior with your goals and values.

Meanwhile, a growing body of research highlights additional health benefits from this metabolic state. For example, a ketogenic diet has shown promises in improving conditions ranging from epilepsy — its original, well-documented use — to Alzheimer's disease, autism, Parkinson's, and even certain forms of cancer. The mechanisms are multifactorial — reduced glucose availability to tumors, reduced neuroinflammation, enhanced neuronal energy production — but all reflect the ability of this diet to profoundly affect physiology at a deep level.

Some people find their mental clarity and focus improving on a ketogenic diet. This phenomenon — sometimes called "keto clarity"— likely results from the brain's ability to use ketones more efficiently than glucose under certain conditions. Ketones produce more energy per molecule of oxygen and generate less reactive oxygen species — in other words, less metabolic waste — which may translate into clearer thinking and less neuronal stress. Furthermore, this state dampens fluctuations in neuronal energy supply, making the brain less prone to dysfunction and more resilient under stress.

CHAPTER 3 — THE SCIENCE OF FAT ADAPTATION

When we talk about the science of fat adaptation, we're really describing a remarkable transformation — a profound metabolic shift — that occurs when you move away from a carbohydrate-centric diet and allow your body to become proficient at using a different, more enduring, and more efficient energy source. Naturally, the human body has a strong preference for glucose under ordinary conditions. Glucose is a quick, easily accessible form of energy — a kind of metabolic fast food — that can be burned quickly and efficiently when it's available in abundance. Whenever you consume carbohydrates — whether from a warm loaf of bread, a bowl of rice, a plate of creamy pasta, a piece of fruit, or a rich dessert — your digestive system converts those carbohydrates into glucose. That glucose enters your bloodstream and signals your pancreas to release insulin, a powerful storage and signaling hormone designed to move glucose into your cells and dampen the release of energy from your own stores.

This process made perfect sense in an ancestral context. There were periods when food was abundant — when the trees were heavy with fruit, when roots were plentiful, or when a successful hunt provided a rich meal — and the body could temporarily rely on a rich carbohydrate intake. There were also periods of scarcity, when carbohydrates were hard to come by. So our physiology is designed to be flexible — able to use whatever energy sources are available. Nonetheless, in modern society, we typically eat carbohydrate-rich foods all day long — a bowl of cereal in the morning, a sandwich at lunch, a plate of pasta at dinner — and this constant delivery of glucose dampens the signals for our body to become proficient at using its own stores of energy.

This is where a ketogenic diet, and the subsequent process of becoming fat-adaptation, comes into play. When you cut back dramatically on carbohydrate intake — dropping it to 20–50 grams per day — you withdraw that reliable stream of glucose. Suddenly, your body finds itself in a predicament: it must find a new way to produce energy. Your pancreas starts to release less insulin, reflecting the lower glucose entering your blood. This drop in insulin signals your body to release fatty acids from its own storage — mainly from your adipose (fat) tissue — into your circulation.

Your liver then converts these fatty acids into small molecules called ketone bodies — acetoacetate, beta-hydroxybutyrate, and a small amount of acetone — which become a powerful and viable energy source for nearly all the cells in your body. Your muscles, your heart, and even your brain — which normally rely nearly exclusively on glucose — learn to use these ketone bodies efficiently. Meanwhile, your mitochondria — the tiny powerhouses within your cells — start to upregulate the production of the enzyme and transport mechanisms needed to efficiently break down fatty acids and ketones for energy.

This process involves a dramatic shift in your metabolic machinery. Certain genes that were previously less active become upregulated, turning on a suite of proteins designed for fatty acid oxidation and ketone utilization. Meanwhile, the genes responsible for carbohydrate utilization diminish in activity, reflecting your body's reduced dependence on glucose.

This transformation typically occurs over a period of 2–4 weeks. During this adaptation, many people experience temporary symptoms — often called the "keto flu"— which can manifest as weakness, headaches, muscle cramps, and a feeling of lethargy. These symptoms reflect your body's ongoing adjustment, as its enzyme systems and metabolic pathways reorganize to accommodate this new way of fueling itself. It's a bit like a factory undergoing a dramatic retool — temporarily messy and inefficient — but once the new production lines are up and running smoothly, the results are dramatic.

Your energy becomes more stable and sustained. Instead of experiencing dramatic drops in energy between carbohydrate-rich meals — drops that typically manifest as "crashed" energy and persistent hunger — your body now has a vast reserve of energy in its own fat stores. This means you can draw upon those reserves at a slow, steady rate, without needing constant refueling from food. Your physical and mental performance become more consistent, your ability to concentrate and focus for extended periods improves, and many people report a newfound clarity of thought — a phenomenon sometimes called "keto clarity."

Your hunger signals diminish because your body is no longer battling fluctuations in glucose and insulin. Instead, the slow, sustained release of fatty acids and ketone bodies provides a stable flow of energy. This stability signals to your hunger centers in the brain — particularly the hypothalamus — that there's no crisis or scarcity, reducing the drive to eat frequently. This, in turn, makes it much easier to follow a ketogenic diet over the long term, without feeling deprived or obsessed with food.

Meanwhile, numerous health benefits emerge from this metabolic state. Your blood sugar drops and stabilises, reducing the risk of diabetes and improving symptoms in those who already suffer from the disease. Your insulin drops, reflecting a lower need for this storage and signaling hormone. Your triglycerides diminish, HDL (the "good") cholesterol often increases, and small dense LDL particles — strongly associated with atherosclerosis — typically diminish.

Your body starts reducing excess water retention and chronic inflammation — two contributors to a range of health disorders. Furthermore, your muscles become proficient at conserving their own proteins and amino acids during this state. This means that you predominantly lose body fat while retaining lean muscle, a phenomenon that makes ketogenic dieting an effective tool for improving body composition. Your body finds a perfect metabolic balance — consuming its own excess while preserving what it needs most.

Meanwhile, this state profoundly influences your physiology at a deep, cellular level. Your mitochondria become more numerous and more efficient. Your body signals for the production of additional mitochondrial components, a process called mitochondrial biogenesis. This means you are not just shifting the energy you use — you are strengthening the powerhouses of your cells — adding depth and resiliency to your metabolic health.

Your ability to perform physical activity, whether it's sustained jogging or heavy lifting, is supported by a well-fueled, adaptable energy system. Your muscles can produce energy efficiently for longer periods, without the dramatic drops in performance that typically come from depleted glycogen stores. This phenomenon has made ketogenic dieting popular amongst athletes — particularly those participating in ultra-endurance events — who appreciate a reliable, nearly inexhaustible energy supply from their own body's resources.

Meanwhile, your brain, which normally relies predominantly on glucose, starts to use ketone bodies, particularly beta-hydroxybutyrate, as a primary energy substrate. This is a dramatic shift in neuronal physiology. Ketone utilization by the brain has numerous benefits — it produces less reactive oxygen species during energy production, yielding a "cleaner" form of energy, and it dampens neuronal hyperexcitability, which is helpful in conditions like epilepsy and neurodegenerative disorders. Some people find their ability to concentrate and perform mentally under stress improves once their brains become proficient at using ketones.

This highlights a key principle of human physiology — adaptability. Your body is designed to respond to changing conditions, whether it's scarcity or abundance. Ketogenic dieting simply signals your physiology to activate a set of genes, enzymes, and metabolic pathways that were always there, waiting to be called upon. This ability reflects an ancient survival mechanism — a way to cope during periods of famine or scarcity — but now we can leverage it to combat a modern lifestyle filled with excess and metabolic dysfunction.

What is especially fascinating about fat adaptation is how it changes the very rhythm of your daily existence. Before this shift, many people feel tethered to a cycle of constant eating. They wake up hungry, reach for breakfast, and then find themselves needing snacks or a large lunch just to keep their energy stable. By mid-afternoon, they might experience that familiar crash — the dip in energy that sends them hunting for coffee, sweets, or other quick fixes. This is the hallmark of a metabolism dependent on glucose — it constantly demands external input to keep blood sugar stable, and any lapse leads to fatigue, irritability, or cravings.

But once your body becomes fat-adapted, you notice that these constant signals of hunger and energy dips begin to fade. There is no longer that urgent need to "top up" your fuel tank every few hours. Instead, your body effortlessly taps into its own fat stores, burning them steadily and smoothly. The result is that you feel lighter, clearer, and more in control. Many people report that they can skip meals without noticing, or go through busy days without being distracted by hunger. This isn't because they are suppressing hunger through sheer willpower — it's because the metabolic processes that trigger those hunger signals have quieted down.

Fat adaptation also offers a unique form of resilience. In a glucose-dependent state, missing a meal can feel like a crisis. Blood sugar drops, and the body responds by releasing stress hormones like cortisol and adrenaline to compensate. This can leave you feeling anxious, shaky, or irritable. But in a fat-adapted state, missing a meal is no crisis at all. Your body simply shifts to burning a little more fat, and you carry on with steady energy and a clear mind. This metabolic flexibility — the ability to smoothly transition between fed and fasted states — is one of the great gifts of fat adaptation.

At the cellular level, this shift brings about remarkable changes. The mitochondria in your cells, which are responsible for producing energy, begin to function more efficiently. They burn fatty acids and ketone bodies in a way that generates less waste, in the form of reactive oxygen species, than burning glucose does. This means that your cells experience less oxidative stress, which is a key factor in aging and in many chronic diseases. Over time, this reduction in oxidative damage supports healthier tissues, whether in your heart, your liver, your brain, or your muscles.

Furthermore, fat adaptation leads to changes in hormone levels that support long-term health. Your insulin levels remain low and stable, reducing the signals to store fat and reducing the risk of insulin resistance — a key factor in the development of type 2 diabetes. Your levels of glucagon, the hormone that signals fat breakdown, rise to support fat burning. Leptin and ghrelin, the hormones that regulate hunger and satiety, begin to shift in a way that promotes natural appetite control. You no longer feel driven by cravings or by the compulsion to eat more than you need.

These hormonal shifts also affect inflammation, one of the silent drivers of chronic disease. Chronic high insulin levels and high blood sugar promote inflammation at the cellular level. This inflammation contributes to a range of conditions, from cardiovascular disease to joint pain to neurodegenerative disorders. But when you're fat-adapted, and your blood sugar and insulin are low and stable, inflammatory markers in your body typically decrease. Many people notice this in the form of reduced joint pain, clearer skin, better digestion, or an overall sense of wellness.

The mental benefits of fat adaptation are equally profound. The brain is a remarkably energy-hungry organ, consuming about 20% of the body's total energy even though it represents only about 2% of body weight. In a fat-adapted state, the brain receives a steady supply of ketones, which are a cleaner, more efficient fuel source. Ketones provide more energy per molecule of oxygen consumed than glucose does, which means the brain operates more efficiently. People often describe a sense of mental clarity, sharper focus, and enhanced memory. For some, this is one of the most motivating aspects of the ketogenic lifestyle — the feeling of being fully awake, alert, and capable.

This mental clarity isn't just a subjective feeling; it reflects real changes in brain chemistry and function. Ketones reduce the excitability of neurons, which is one reason why the ketogenic diet has been so effective for controlling epilepsy. They also reduce oxidative stress in the brain, support the growth of new neuronal connections, and may protect against the neurodegeneration seen in conditions like Alzheimer's disease. Emerging research even suggests that a ketogenic state can improve mood and reduce symptoms of anxiety and depression — likely because of these stabilizing and protective effects on brain function.

The journey to fat adaptation does require patience and persistence. During the initial weeks, as your body makes the shift, you might experience fatigue, lightheadedness, or cravings — what's commonly called the keto flu. This isn't a sign of harm; it's a sign that your body is recalibrating. You can support this transition by staying hydrated, ensuring adequate intake of electrolytes like sodium, potassium, and magnesium, and allowing your body time to adjust. As the weeks pass, these symptoms fade, and you find yourself feeling stronger and more vibrant than before.

Once fully fat-adapted, you'll notice that your performance in physical activities may actually improve. Endurance athletes, in particular, benefit from fat adaptation because it provides a nearly limitless source of fuel. Where glucose stores might run out after a couple of hours of activity, fat stores can sustain the body for much longer. This is why many ultra-endurance athletes have turned to ketogenic diets to help them perform at their best without relying on constant intake of carbohydrate gels or drinks.

Your body composition also reflects these changes. Fat adaptation supports the loss of body fat while preserving lean muscle mass. Because insulin levels stay low, your body isn't driven to store excess calories as fat. At the same time, the preservation of muscle is supported by ketones themselves, which have been shown to have a muscle-sparing effect. This makes fat adaptation an excellent strategy not just for weight loss but for building a stronger, more functional body.

As you move further into fat adaptation, you begin to experience the full spectrum of its benefits. Your digestion may improve, with less bloating or discomfort after meals. Your sleep may become deeper and more restful, as blood sugar fluctuations that disrupt sleep cycles are minimized. Your immune function may strengthen, thanks to lower inflammation and improved nutrient absorption. Even your skin may appear healthier, reflecting the internal improvements in oxidative stress and inflammation.

Ultimately, fat adaptation represents a return to a more natural, ancestral way of fueling the body. For much of human history, people lived in conditions where carbohydrates were not always abundant. Our bodies evolved to thrive on fat as a primary fuel source during these times. By adopting a ketogenic diet and becoming fat-adapted, you are tapping into this ancient wisdom — allowing your body to function in the way it was designed. You are reclaiming metabolic flexibility, restoring balance to your hormones, and creating a foundation for lifelong health and vitality.

CHAPTER 4 — BENEFIT BREAKDOWN

When you embark upon a ketogenic lifestyle, you are not simply following another diet — you are igniting a deep, profound transformation within your body. It's a transformation that starts at a cellular level and ripples upward through nearly every aspect of your health and well-being. To appreciate just how powerful this process can be, we need to move away from the view that food is a collection of calories and macronutrients. Instead, we should view it as information — signals — messages that we send directly to our physiology. A ketogenic diet is a powerful message. It tells your body to shift from a state of storage and dependence on a steady stream of carbohydrates and glucose to a state of liberation — a state in which your body starts drawing upon its own abundant energy stores.

Weight loss is often the first dramatic result people notice. There's a very clear, logical physiology underpinning this phenomenon. Traditionally, when we consume a diet rich in carbohydrates, our pancreas responds by releasing insulin, a powerful storage hormone. The main role of insulin is to clear excess glucose from the blood and move it into cells. But under a ketogenic diet, carbohydrate intake drops profoundly, which means the stimulus for insulin release drops alongside it. As a result, your body finds it can no longer rely on a constant infusion of glucose for energy. Instead, it starts to break down stored body fat into fatty acids and converts them into ketone bodies — a clean, efficient energy that muscles and the brain can readily use.

This metabolic shift from a glucose-dependent state to a fat-fueled state signals your body to let go of its excess reserves. Naturally, over days and weeks, you will observe a reduction in body-fat percentages and a trimming of the waistline. Importantly, this isn't just a temporary phenomenon; it's a sustained, deep change — a dramatic reshaping — made possible by a fundamental metabolic reprogramming.

As your body grows more proficient at accessing its own fat stores, another remarkable process occurs: your blood sugar and insulin levels stabilize. The dramatic fluctuations — the "crashed" feeling after a carbohydrate-heavy meal — diminish. Without large surges in glucose entering your circulation, your pancreas isn't constantly called upon to release large amounts of insulin. Your cells become more sensitive to the small amounts of insulin you do produce. That means your body regains its ability to regulate its own energy gracefully and efficiently, reducing your risk of developing Type 2 diabetes.

This reduction in glucose and insulin signals has a dramatic ripple effect across many aspects of health. Your HDL — often called "the good cholesterol"— typically increases, reflecting improved lipid transport and reduced cardiovascular risk. Simultanously, your LDL and triglycerides diminish. Elevated LDL and triglycerides are well-documented contributors to atherosclerosis and heart disease. So this favorable shift in your lipid profile signals a move toward greater cardiovascular health — a literal renewal of your arterial health.

Some people report a dramatic reduction in chronic inflammation and joint pain after adopting a ketogenic diet. There are numerous mechanisms at play here. Elevated glucose and insulin promote the production of pro-inflammatory cytokines — signaling molecules that activate the body's stress responses. Furthermore, excess carbohydrate consumption can contribute to the formation of advanced glycation end products (AGEs), compounds that damage proteins and tissues and exacerbate chronic pain and dysfunction. By reducing carbohydrate intake and shifting to a state of metabolic flexibility, you dampen these pro-inflammatory signals. Your body finds a new peace, a state of reduced chronic stress — which many people experience as less joint pain and a greater ease of movement in their daily lives.

Some individuals find the ketogenic diet helpful in managing conditions like epilepsy, polycystic ovary syndrome (PCOS), and metabolic syndrome — disorders that all have roots in metabolic dysfunction. The neuroprotective effects of ketone bodies, particularly beta-hydroxybutyrate, have been recognized for nearly a century in the context of epilepsy, where a ketogenic diet can reduce the frequency of seizures in children and adults who are medication-resistant. Women with PCOS, a condition strongly associated with insulin resistance, often find their symptoms diminish when carbohydrate intake drops and insulin resistance improves. Metabolic syndrome — a collection of abnormalities including elevated glucose, high triglycerides, low HDL, and abdominal obesity — responds profoundly to carbohydrate reduction, reflecting the ability of a ketogenic diet to attack its root cause.

Some research also suggests ketogenic diets may be protective against neurodegenerative disorders — Alzheimer's, Parkinson's, and related conditions — by reducing neuronal stress and improving energy delivery to the brain. The human brain normally relies nearly exclusively on glucose for energy. But when ketones are present, the brain can efficiently use them as an alternative, protective energy source. Furthermore, a growing body of research highlights ketone bodies' ability to reduce oxidative stress, dampen neuroinflammation, and promote neuronal health — mechanisms that collectively help to safeguard the brain against age-related disorders.

Your daily energy, mood, and mental clarity frequently improve on a ketogenic diet. Without dramatic fluctuations in glucose, your energy delivery becomes more stable and sustained. The "fog" and "crashed" feeling many people associate with drops in blood sugar diminish, yielding a sense of clarity and focus. Furthermore, ketone bodies provide a more efficient form of energy for the brain; for many, this results in sharper thinking, enhanced productivity, and a more stable mood.

Ultimately, a ketogenic diet transforms health at a deep, fundamental level. It signals your body to move away from a state of storage and dependency toward a state of metabolic flexibility and renewal. The result is not just a thinner waistline or lower number on a scale — it's a dramatic improvement in health across numerous dimensions. Your body finds its native ability to regulate energy, to heal, to reduce inflammation, and to optimize its own physiology. The benefits ripple through nearly every aspect of health — from your metabolic health to your neurobiology — reflecting a powerful transformation made possible by a simple but profound change in diet.

As this transformation unfolds, something remarkable starts to happen — you become more in tune with your body's signals. The cravings for processed carbohydrates diminish. Your energy, once prone to dramatic drops and surges, finds a new baseline of stability. Naturally, you find yourself feeling more satiated after a meal rich in healthy fats and proteins. There's a newfound peace with food; it no longer exerts power over you in the form of cravings, temptation, or persistent hunger signals. Instead of battling your willpower all day, you realize you simply aren't thinking about food nearly as much. Your body has become proficient at accessing its own stores when it needs energy, making you less prone to snacking and binge-eating.

This reduced drive to eat frequently — sometimes called "food freedom" — is a dramatic shift for many people who have previously felt enslaved by their appetites. It signals a return to a more natural way of relating to food, a state in which you eat when you're hungry and stop when you're full. Importantly, this change in behavior isn't something you're forcing upon yourself; it's a direct result of your physiology shifting toward a state of metabolic health.

This newfound freedom from persistent hunger makes it much easier to maintain a calorie deficit when you need to lose weight, and it makes it less likely that you'll suffer from rebound weight gain — a phenomenon frequently called "yo-yo dieting"— which occurs when restrictive diets undermine your metabolic health and drive you back toward over-eating once you revert to your normal habits.

Meanwhile, a cascade of health benefits you may not immediately see is underway beneath the surface. Your pancreas is experiencing a much-needed rest from its constant output of insulin. Your liver, which plays a key role in converting excess glucose into triglycerides and storing it in fatty deposits, starts to clear its own fatty stores — a process known as reducing fatty liver. The improvement in liver health has numerous ripple effects across your physiology, influencing everything from your ability to regulate blood sugar to your production of essential proteins and components for proper detoxification.

Your muscles become more proficient at burning fatty acids and ketone bodies for energy, reducing their reliance on glucose and improving their metabolic flexibility. At the same time, your mitochondria — the tiny powerhouses within your cells — become more numerous and more efficient. The result is a dramatic improvement in physical and mental energy, a renewal at the cellular level. Your ability to perform daily tasks, pursue physical activity, and concentrate on challenging mental tasks all improve.

This renewal extends to your cardiovascular health in profoundly protective ways. Large fluctuations in glucose and insulin can damage the delicate endothelial cells that line your arteries, making it more likely for plaque to form and atherosclerosis to progress. By stabilizing these fluctuations and reducing chronic inflammation, a ketogenic diet assists your body in healing these injured areas and improving arterial health. Your risk of developing cardiovascular disease drops in a way that's measurable — in your blood work and in your physical fitness — reflecting the powerful, multi-layered benefits of this lifestyle.

For many, this transformation underscores a dramatic reversal of a trajectory toward poor health. Metabolic syndrome — a condition defined by abdominal obesity, elevated glucose, high blood pressure, abnormal lipid profiles, and reduced HDL — often responds profoundly to a ketogenic diet. The components of this syndrome collectively raise the risk for Type 2 diabetes, heart disease, stroke, and other chronic disorders. But when you cut carbohydrate intake and allow your body to become proficient at burning its own fatty deposits for energy, these abnormalities frequently resolve, sometimes in a matter of weeks or months.

This resolution signals more than just an improvement in health; it highlights a deep, fundamental healing — a return to metabolic health. Your body is designed to regulate itself gracefully when given the proper signals, and a ketogenic diet provides exactly those signals.

Meanwhile, a growing body of research underscores protective effects against neurodegenerative disorders. Scientists are investigating how ketone bodies, particularly beta-hydroxybutyrate, can act as an alternative energy substrate for neuronal cells when glucose utilization is impaired, as it often is in conditions like Alzheimer's Disease. Furthermore, ketone bodies may help reduce the production of reactive oxygen species — damaging compounds that contribute to neuronal dysfunction — and dampen neuroinflammation, a key process in the progression of disorders like Alzheimer's, Parkinson's, and multiple sclerosis.

Some research even points toward an upregulation of neuroprotective factors and growth signals, suggesting a ketogenic diet may foster neurogenesis — the growth of new neurons — and synaptic renewal. If this is true, it could have dramatic implications not just for slowing disease progression, but for improving neuronal health, memory, and cognitive function.

Meanwhile, the benefits to your mood and mental clarity frequently become a subjective indicator that something powerful is changing within you. People report an ability to concentrate more deeply, a reduction in "foggy thinking", and a greater stability of mood. There's a biochemical basis for these reports. The brain prefers a stable delivery of energy; large fluctuations in glucose can undermine neuronal function and affect the release of key neurochemicals. The ketogenic diet provides a more stable, sustained energy flow to the brain, and this stability is believed to be responsible for many of the subjective improvements in mood and clarity.

Furthermore, reduced chronic inflammation — a state strongly influenced by diet — may allow the nervous system to operate more efficiently. Certain proinflammatory cytokines can affect neuroplasticity, undermine synaptic health, and diminish neuronal communication. By reducing these signals, a ketogenic diet may help the nervous system repair itself and foster a more robust, adaptable network of communication — a phenomenon that underpins learning, memory, and overall mental health.

CHAPTER 5 — MYTHS AND MISCONCEPTIONS

When you first embark upon a ketogenic lifestyle, it's not unusual to encounter a chorus of doubts, misconceptions, and myths — many stemming from years of misinformation and a fundamental misunderstanding of human physiology. The ketogenic diet has become a powerful tool for health transformation, yet it's frequently dismissed as a dangerous "fad diet" or misunderstood by those who haven't taken the time to appreciate its rich history, its strong scientific foundations, and its remarkable ability to heal. So in this chapter, we're going to cut through the confusion. We're going to illuminate the facts, dismantling the myths piece by piece, and empowering you to move forward with confidence, understanding, and a clear view of what this lifestyle really means.

To appreciate this fully, we need to start by addressing the most persistent and pervasive myth — that the ketogenic diet is some kind of dangerous or unreliable "fad." The reality is quite the opposite. There is nothing faddish about a way of eating that has roots deep in human physiology and a rich, documented history in medicine. The ketogenic diet traces back nearly a century to its use in epilepsy treatment, particularly for children who were not responsive to medication. Scientists and doctors recognized that when carbohydrate intake drops and the body starts to produce ketone bodies for energy, seizures often diminish or resolve altogether. That observation opened the door to decades of research into how a state of nutritional ketosis — far from being a health hazard — can be profoundly healing.

This rich history underscores a key point: ketogenic eating isn't a diet trend; it's a well-established, physiologically grounded approach to health. The human body has a remarkable ability to produce its own glucose and energy from fatty acids and ketone bodies when carbohydrate intake drops. We carry this ability within us because it provided a survival advantage for our ancestors during periods of scarcity, when food was unreliable and carbohydrate-rich sources were scarce. So when we say we are entering a state of ketosis, we are not forcing something abnormal upon our physiology; we are reconnecting with a metabolic path that has supported human health and survival for millennia.

Some people say we need carbohydrates for energy — ignoring the body's ability to produce its own glucose and to efficiently utilize ketone bodies. Naturally, under a carbohydrate-rich diet, the body predominantly relies on glucose for energy. But when carbohydrate intake drops, a metabolic shift occurs. The liver converts fatty acids into ketone bodies — primarily beta-hydroxybutyrate and acetoacetate — which become a potent, clean, and efficient energy source for nearly all tissues, including the brain. Furthermore, for those few cells in the body that require glucose, the liver can produce it from non-carbohydrate sources through a process called gluconeogenesis. So we are never entirely without glucose; the body simply makes what it needs.

This ability underscores a key principle — we are not dependent on a constant supply of carbohydrates. Our physiology is designed to be flexible, adaptive, and proficient at accessing a range of energy sources. To say we "need" carbohydrates disregards this adaptability and the metabolic prowess we possess.

Another frequently misunderstood notion is that a ketogenic diet is all about "eating bacon"— or gorging on processed meats and poor sources of fats. That view comes from a simplistic view of macronutrients and disregards the rich, whole foods that form the basis of a well-formulated ketogenic diet. Naturally raised meats, fatty fish rich in omega-3s, avocado, olives, coconut oil, and a vast array of non-starchy vegetables all have a place in this way of eating. The emphasis is on choosing whole, nutrient-dense foods — not processed products — and designing a plate rich in healthy fats, abundant in vitamins and antioxidants, and low in carbohydrate. The result is a diet that nourishes at a deep level, delivering a range of nutrients while keeping carbohydrate intake to a minimum.

Some fear this diet will raise their cholesterol and undermine their health, ignoring extensive research that shows health markers typically improve on a ketogenic diet. HDL, the "good" cholesterol, often increases; LDL particles become large and fluffy — a pattern associated with lower cardiovascular risk; and triglycerides diminish, reflecting a dramatic improvement in metabolic health. Furthermore, numerous studies show reductions in chronic inflammation and markers of metabolic dysfunction. The narrative that consuming healthy fats is hazardous simply disregards this growing body of evidence — and it fails to appreciate the context. Our health is influenced by numerous factors, not just total cholesterol; a rich view must account for particle size, HDL, triglycerides, and the context of diet and lifestyle.

Some say the ketogenic diet is hard to follow — restrictive, challenging, or socially isolating — but this view disregards the power of meal planning, education, and preparation. Naturally, when we first move away from a diet we're accustomed to, it can feel challenging. There may be a period of adaptation — often called the "keto flu"— when the body adjusts its enzyme production and starts making greater use of fatty acids and ketone bodies. But this is a temporary phenomenon. With proper education, meal plans, and support, most people find the diet not only doable but profoundly satisfying and liberating. They appreciate the reduced cravings, the freedom from constant hunger, and the ability to enjoy rich, savory foods without guilt. Furthermore, a growing community of resources — from blogs and cookbooks to online groups — makes it easier than ever to find meal ideas, troubleshoot obstacles, and connect with others on a similar path.

Some confuse ketogenic with Atkins or Paleo, failing to appreciate the key distinctions. Atkins typically starts with a dramatic reduction in carbohydrates but then reintroduces them in phases. Paleo focuses on whole, unprocessed foods in a way that broadly resembles a hunter-gatherer diet. Keto, by contrast, maintains a low carbohydrate intake to keep the body in a state of nutritional ketosis, emphasizing a diet rich in healthy fats. Each approach has its benefits, but ketogenic is unique in its ability to induce and maintain ketosis — a metabolic state that profoundly influences energy production, disease risk, and overall health.

This chapter aims to clear up confusion and empower you with knowledge. There's a dramatic transformation available to you if you can cut through the myths and appreciate the rich, powerful physiology of this diet. A ketogenic lifestyle isn't a fad; it's a well-established, well-studied path to health — a path designed by nature and supported by a growing body of scientific and clinical data.

With the myths gone, you can move forward with confidence and understanding. You can appreciate this diet not as a restrictive regimen, but as a powerful tool for healing and renewal — a way to reconnect with your body's native ability to generate energy, regulate itself, and flourish. The ketogenic diet isn't about following a rigid set of rules; it's about honoring physiology and choosing foods that align with our metabolic design. It's a way to cut through confusion, to find health and happiness from within.

As we move forward and clear away these misconceptions, it's worth pausing to appreciate just how much misinformation has gotten in the way of understanding this way of eating. The diet industry is awash with conflicting messages, many of which are influenced more by marketing trends and agricultural policy than by physiology or health outcomes. The ketogenic diet, by contrast, cuts through the noise by honoring the body's natural ability to produce energy, heal, and maintain health when provided with the appropriate conditions.

Some people fear that reducing carbohydrate intake will undermine physical performance, particularly for athletes. But this view disregards a growing body of research and a multitude of elite athletes who have successfully transitioned to a ketogenic diet — from ultra-marathon runners and triathletes to powerlifters and professional soccer players. Once their bodies become proficient at utilizing fatty acids and ketone bodies for energy — a process called "fat adaptation"— many find their endurance, recovery, and power output improve. They become less reliant on frequent carbohydrate intake, suffer from less "bonking" or energy drops, and enjoy more stable energy levels during extended physical activity.

This phenomenon highlights a key principle: the human body is designed to perform under a range of conditions, provided it has a reliable and efficient energy source. The ability to tap into nearly unlimited stores of body fat and generate energy from it, without needing a constant infusion of carbohydrate, is a powerful metabolic advantage — and it can be a game-changer for athletes and non-athletes alike.

Furthermore, this view underscores another misconception — that a ketogenic diet must undermine muscle mass or lead to muscle wasting. The reality is quite the opposite. The combination of low carbohydrate intake and proper protein consumption signals the body to spare muscle while accessing stored fatty acids for energy. Furthermore, ketone bodies may have a muscle-sparing, "anti-catabolic" effect, reducing the breakdown of muscle proteins under stress. So instead of causing weakness or wasting, a well-formulated ketogenic diet can help maintain or even improve muscle mass and physical performance.

Some people say a ketogenic diet is hard to maintain in a social context — dining with friends, attending parties, or choosing from menus in restaurants. But this view underestimates the adaptability of this lifestyle and the growing awareness and accommodations available in restaurants and grocery stores. It's now easier than ever to find low carbohydrate options on menus and to make substitutions to align a meal with ketogenic guidelines. Grilled proteins, salads tossed in olive oil, avocado-rich dishes, and creamy sauces made from healthful fats are frequently available — and these choices allow you to stay true to your diet while participating in social events and communal dining. Furthermore, when you appreciate this diet not as a temporary "quick-fix" but as a way of life, these choices become effortless, and you naturally gravitate toward foods and menus that nourish you and align with your goals.

Some confuse ketogenic with restrictive, boring, or overly restrictive, ignoring the rich array of foods available — from fatty cuts of meat, seafood, and full-fat dairy to non-starchy vegetables, avocado, olives, and a whole world of herbs and seasonings. Furthermore, a burgeoning market of low carbohydrate ingredients — from nut flours and alternative sweeteners to specialty products — makes it easier than ever to create a rich, satisfying ketogenic plate. The result is a diet that feels indulgent, not restrictive — a diet that you can enjoy day in and day out without feeling deprived.

Meanwhile, this lifestyle can profoundly affect not just physical health but mental health and well-being. There is a growing understanding of the relationship between diet, inflammation, and disorders of the mind — from autism and Alzheimer's to depression and anxiety. The ketogenic diet has a powerful anti-inflammatory effect and can affect neurochemistry in ways that promote stability and clarity. Furthermore, by stabilizing glucose and reducing fluctuations in blood sugar and insulin, the diet may help to ease the symptoms of disorders influenced by metabolic dysfunction in the brain. There is a growing body of research investigating ketogenic therapies for conditions ranging from bipolar disorder to autism spectrum disorders, adding a rich and hopeful dimension to its health benefits.

Some people say "ketogenic isn't for everyone"— and there's a kernel of truth in this. Certain health conditions — such as disorders of fatty acid oxidation or certain metabolic disorders — may prohibit a person from safely entering a state of ketosis. Furthermore, medication regimes, health conditions, and individual preferences must be taken into account when designing a diet. That's why it's always recommended to seek guidance from a health professional who is well-versed in ketogenic therapy and can help customize an approach to match an individual's needs.

But these cases are the exception, not the rule. The vast majority of people can safely and effectively follow a well-formulated ketogenic diet and experience dramatic health improvements. Importantly, this isn't a "one-size-fits-all" approach — there's a spectrum of carbohydrate intake, a range of food choices, and numerous strategies for tailoring a ketogenic lifestyle to an individual's preferences and health goals. The key is education, understanding, and willingness to learn and adapt.

The ketogenic diet, then, isn't a restrictive diet in the punitive sense — it's a powerful tool for transformation. It's a path back toward metabolic health, a way to align your physiology with its designed state of functionality. It clears away the confusion stemming from misinformation and diet fads, and it provides a clear, actionable framework for health.

CHAPTER 6 — MEASURING SUCCESS

As you progress on your ketogenic journey, it's crucial to appreciate that true success isn't defined by a number on a scale alone. Your transformation is a rich, multi-layered process — a metamorphosis — that permeates nearly every aspect of health and well-being. Measuring success means looking at a range of indicators, not just your weight, to appreciate the full picture of your progress. It means honoring all the signals your body is sending you — signals that reflect metabolic health, energy, mood, physical performance, and a newfound sense of control over your lifestyle. Success, in this context, is not a destination defined by a single number; it's a rich, ongoing journey toward health, resiliency, and renewal.

Your scale can certainly be a helpful tool. It can track trends in your body weight over time and reflect broad patterns — whether you're losing excess body fat or retaining water. But a scale simply reports total mass; it can't tell you about your body composition — how much of you is muscle, how much is water, and how much is body fat. Furthermore, numerous factors can affect your scale weight from day to day — sodium intake, hydration, stress, and the time of day — making it an unreliable gauge when viewed in isolation. That's why we need additional measures to illuminate the true progress you're making.

This is where body measurements come into play. Measuring your waist, hips, thighs, and arms regularly — say once a week or once a month — can be a powerful way to track physical change. Often, you will find that you're losing inches and dropping sizes even if your scale isn't reflecting dramatic drops in weight. That's because muscle is denser than fat, and your body may be reshaping itself in a way that the scale simply can't show. If you were previously retaining water or experiencing bloating and now you're losing excess fluids, or swapping body fat for muscle, your measurements will reflect those subtler — yet profoundly important — transforms.

Body-fat percentage is another key indicator of progress. Techniques like skinfold calipers, bioelectrical impedance, or DEXA scans can give you a more accurate view of your body's composition. Ideally, you want to aim for a gradual reduction in body-fat while retaining or even adding muscle. A drop in body-fat is a clear sign you're tapping into your body's ability to use its own stores for energy — a main objective of a ketogenic lifestyle. Importantly, this process underscores health, not just appearance; excess body-fat, particularly visceral fat, is strongly tied to metabolic dysfunction and disease.

For those who appreciate hard data, ketone testing is a powerful way to track whether you're in a state of nutritional ketosis — the metabolic state in which your body is predominantly burning fatty acids and ketone bodies instead of glucose. There are a few methods to test for ketones. Urine test strips, for example, measure acetoacetate, a waste product of ketosis. Although convenient and inexpensive, urine tests become less accurate once you're fully adapted to a ketogenic diet, because your body starts using ketones more efficiently instead of excreting them. At that point, a more precise method — a blood ketone meter — is preferred. It directly measures beta-hydroxybutyrate, the primary ketone in circulation, offering a clear view of whether you're in a state of deep nutritional ketosis.

Non-scale victories — or NSVs — are another profoundly important piece of the progress puzzle. Although hard data is helpful, some of the greatest benefits people report from a ketogenic lifestyle are subjective, lifestyle-related, and sometimes hard to quantify. Rising energy levels, for example, reflect a dramatic shift in your body's ability to produce sustained, stable energy from its own stores, instead of experiencing the dramatic drops and "crashes" associated with a carbohydrate-rich diet. Mood stabilization and reduced cravings for sweets or starchier foods are signals your physiology is becoming less driven by fluctuations in blood sugar and more anchored in a steady, reliable energy state.

Some people find their thinking becomes clearer and more focused, their memory sharper, and their ability to concentrate for extended periods improved. Others appreciate dramatic reductions in joint pain and chronic discomfort, a reflection of reduced inflammation. Better skin, more restful sleep, and greater physical endurance are frequently reported by those following a ketogenic lifestyle. All these subjective indicators reflect deep, metabolic healing — a renewal from the inside out — that often precedes more visible physical change.

Your health markers — your "inner numbers"— can reflect dramatic transformation, even if your physical appearance has not yet completely shifted. Fasting glucose typically drops and stabilises, reflecting improved insulin sensitivity and reduced resistance. Hemoglobin A1c, a measure of average blood glucose over the past two to three months, often falls into a healthy range, reducing your future risk of diabetes and complications. Serum lipids may show improvement in HDL (the "good" cholesterol), a reduction in small, dense LDL particles, and a drop in triglycerides — all signals of reduced cardiovascular risk. Furthermore, blood pressure often normalises, reflecting reduced stiffness in the arteries and a drop in sodium retention — two key components of health and metabolic resiliency.

Fitness performance and recovery can also be a powerful indicator of adaptation. As your body becomes proficient at using fatty acids and ketone bodies for energy, you may find you can perform physical activity with greater ease and for longer periods without needing to refuel frequently. Your recovery from strenuous activity may be quicker, reflecting reduced inflammation and more efficient repair mechanisms. Furthermore, retaining muscle while losing body-fat underscores your ability to maintain, and even improve, physical functionality — a key indicator of health and metabolic stability.

Sleep, stress, and mental clarity — subjective signals — are powerful indicators that your physiology is shifting in a desirable direction. If you find you're falling asleep more easily, staying asleep through the night, and waking feeling rested and clearheaded, it signals your nervous and endocrine systems are achieving a more restful, balanced state. If you find stress feels more manageable and your mood more stable, it may reflect reduced fluctuations in blood sugar and stress hormones, and a more resilient physiology.

Ultimately, it's this combination — scale, measurements, body-fat, health markers, physical performance, subjective well-being — that provides the fullest picture of your progress. Viewing these signals together lets you appreciate health from a 360-degree perspective. It underscores the principle that health is not defined by a single number or a moment in time, but by a rich pattern of improvement across numerous dimensions.

As you progress on this journey, it's crucial to appreciate patience and persistence. Your body is not a machine with an "on/off" button; it's a sophisticated, adaptive system designed to respond and heal in its own time. There will be periods of dramatic change, where progress seems effortless and nearly every measure — from scale to mood — shows improvement. There will be plateaus, where progress appears to slow or even temporarily halt, and that's entirely normal. Your physiology may be busy healing deep-rooted dysfunctions — reducing chronic inflammation, improving mitochondrial health, and strengthening metabolic pathways — and these subtler processes take time.

This highlights the necessity of focusing on lifestyle over short-term fluctuations. Viewing your progress through a multi-faceted lens lets you appreciate the true transformation underway. If you were to rely solely on scale weight, you might become discouraged during a temporary stall — not realizing that, at the same time, your body-fat percentage is dropping, your muscle mass is improving, your energy is more stable, and your health markers are reflecting dramatic internal healing.

Instead of framing progress in black-and-white terms — "I'm losing weight" or "I'm not losing weight" — it's helpful to view health as a spectrum. Each small improvement — a drop in fasting glucose, a rise in HDL, a reduction in waist circumference, more restful nights, less cravings — collectively signals you're headed in a profoundly healthy direction. Small signals add up. They form a rich, multilayered picture of transformation — a picture you will appreciate more and more the further you travel on this path.

Non-scale victories, in particular, illuminate the deep, qualitative dimensions of change. Take, for example, someone who finds their energy is more stable from morning to evening. That signals their body is efficiently generating energy from its own stores instead of experiencing dramatic drops in glucose and subsequent "crashed" energy. That newfound stability translates into greater productivity, clearer thinking, and more patience and peace in daily interactions — benefits that profoundly affect not just physical health, but relationships, work, creativity, and overall happiness.

Another person might find their cravings for sweets diminish, reflecting a dramatic reduction in the neurochemical signals that previously drove a cycle of carbohydrate dependency. That signals a fundamental reprogramming of their physiology — a renewal of metabolic flexibility — which makes future choices profoundly different. Instead of battling temptation or feeling powerless in the face of cravings, they become free to choose foods and habits that align with their goals.

Some find their skin clears, their acne disappears, their hair becomes shinier and their nails grow stronger — signals that deep healing is underway at a cellular level. The reduction in chronic, low-grade inflammation that a ketogenic diet brings can manifest in numerous, sometimes unexpected, ways. Conditions ranging from psoriasis and acne to arthritis and headaches often diminish, reflecting a dramatic reduction in the production of proinflammatory cytokines and other signals of chronic disease.

Meanwhile, many people find their mental health profoundly improves. Mood swings diminish, symptoms of anxiety and depression ease, and there's a newfound clarity and stability in their outlook on life. Some describe it as "having the fog lift"— a dramatic change in their ability to concentrate, remember, and find peace in their daily experience. Certain neurodegenerative disorders, while complex and multi-factorial, may also respond positively to a ketogenic diet, reflecting its ability to reduce neuronal stress and improve energy utilization in the brain.

Fitness and physical performance reflect these internal improvements in dramatic ways. Your ability to perform strenuous activity without "hitting the wall"— a phenomenon well-known to runners and athletes — signals a metabolic shift toward greater fatty acid oxidation and a reduced reliance on limited glycogen stores. Recovery from physical stress, whether from a tough workout or a hectic day, comes more quickly and more completely. Your muscles repair, your nervous system resets, and you find you're ready to perform again without the lingering weakness or stiffness you previously experienced.

Sleep, a key indicator of health, often deepens and becomes more restful once you become proficient at burning fatty acids and ketones for energy. Your body finds its circadian rhythms more stable, your stress physiology settles, and you produce a healthy pulse of melatonin and growth factors overnight — all signals of a body in repair and renewal.

Meanwhile, stress and resiliency — your ability to handle psychological and physical stress — are profoundly influenced by metabolic health. A ketogenic lifestyle dampens the dramatic fluctuations in stress hormones and blood sugar that previously kept you in a state of chronic "fight or flight." Consequently, you become more adaptable, more resilient, more able to handle whatever comes your way. Your nervous system finds a deep peace, and this stability permeates all aspects of your health.

Ultimately, all these signals — scale, measurements, health markers, physical performance, subjective well-being — come together to tell a rich, multilayered story of transformation. It's a story of renewal from the inside out, a story of a body reclaiming its ability to regulate energy, heal, and flourish. Importantly, this renewal occurs not in dramatic, overnight fashion, but through small, persistent, and cumulative change — a testimony to the power of patience, persistence, and honoring the body's innate ability to heal when given the proper conditions.

CHAPTER 7 — YOUR 30-DAY TRANSFORMATION PLAN

Your transformation starts here. It's a powerful moment — a decisive step forward into a new way of living, a new way of honoring and fueling your body. The 30-Day Transformation Plan is more than just a diet; it's a clear, actionable road map to guide you safely, effectively, and gracefully into the metabolic state we call ketosis. It's a state where your body evolves from a sugar-burning machine into a proficient, adaptable, and energetic-fat burner. The path you're about to follow has been carefully crafted to maximize health, minimize discomfort, and produce dramatic results — not just in your physical appearance, but in your energy, mood, and overall well-being.

This transformation is a journey — not a sprint — and the first few days will be an adjustment. Your body has grown comfortable with a carbohydrate-centric diet, and it will need time to learn a new way to produce energy. But rest assured: this is a temporary transition. The first 7–10 days may come with some discomfort — a phenomenon frequently called the "keto flu"— but this is not a true flu; it's simply a sign your body is shifting its metabolic gear. It may manifest in symptoms like headaches, weakness, lethargy, and cravings for carbohydrates. Hydration, proper electrolyte intake, rest, and patience are key during this period, and we'll walk you through exactly how to navigate it safely and effectively.

Your meal plan during these first 30 days will reflect a dramatic reduction in carbohydrate intake — typically dropping to about 20–50 grams per day. Naturally, this signals your body to deplete its stores of glycogen (stored glucose) and to start turning inward — accessing its own fatty acids for energy and ramping up production of ketones in the liver. To facilitate this process, your diet will be rich in healthy fats — avocado, olive oil, fatty fish, grass-fed meats — and will include a moderate amount of high–quality proteins and a small serving of low-starch, fiber-rich veggies. Importantly, you will avoid foods rich in refined carbohydrates — bread, pasta, rice, and sweets — and will instead nourish yourself with whole, unprocessed foods that align with your body's ancestral physiology.

This gradual reduction in carbohydrate is purposeful; it eases you into a state of ketosis without causing needless shock to your system. Ideally, you will cut back your carbohydrate intake over a few days instead of dropping it all at once. Begin by eliminating soda, sweets, and processed foods, then gradually reduce starchy carbohydrates. If you normally eat 200 grams of carbohydrate a day, consider dropping it to 100 grams for a few days, then 50 grams, and then 20–30 grams. This gradual reduction lets your body adjust its enzyme production and metabolic pathways more smoothly, reducing symptoms of the "keto flu."

Your meal plan will reflect this process. The first few days may allow for small amounts of carbohydrate from non-starchy veggies — a handful of strawberries, a serving of zucchini or peppers — alongside a greater emphasis on healthy fats and proteins. Naturally, this ratio will shift toward greater-fat and lower-carbohydrate choices by the second or third week. Your plate might feature fatty cuts of grass-fed steak, wild-caught fatty fish like salmon, avocado-rich salads tossed in olive oil, omelets made with pastured eggs and cheddar, and rich, creamy sauces made from pure heavy cream and herbs. There's an abundance of delicious food available to you — this is not a diet of deprivation, but a rich and satisfying way of eating.

Your daily goals during this 30-Day Transformation will help keep you motivated and on track. Each day you will aim to stay within your carbohydrate limit — typically under 50 grams — while meeting your calorie and macronutrient goals. The meal plan provided in this book will do much of this heavy lifting for you, offering you a clear road map to follow. Daily goals might include consuming at least 2–3 servings of non-starchy veggies, drinking enough fluids and adding a small amount of sodium and potassium to account for losses through urine, and honoring your body's signals — resting when you're fatigued and not overtraining in the gym.

Activity during the first 30 days should be kept light to medium, allowing your body to devote its resources to metabolic adaptation and healing. Your muscles are shifting their preferred energy substrate from glucose to fatty acids and ketones; this process temporarily dampens physical performance and recovery. Activities such as walking, gentle yoga, light resistance training, or short, low-intensity sessions are appropriate during this period. Your main objective during this time is not to conquer heavy weights or pursue strenuous physical goals, but to allow your body to become proficient at a fundamentally different way of fueling itself. Once you're fully adapted, typically after a few weeks, you will find your physical performance rebounding, often exceeding your previous capabilities.

Hydration and electrolyte intake are key components during this period. As you cut back on carbohydrates, your body will release a significant amount of water and sodium — a phenomenon called natriuresis — which can affect your hydration and electrolyte balance. To combat this, you should drink plenty of fluids, aim for at least 2–3 litres per day, and consider adding a small amount of sodium, potassium, and magnesium to your diet to ease symptoms of "keto flu." Foods rich in these nutrients — avocado for potassium, bone broth for sodium, and dark leafy veggies for magnesium — can help you maintain balance and avoid side effects.

Your 30-Day Transformation calendar will outline exactly what you should do each day — what to eat, how much, and when — to maximize your progress. Each day is a small, purposeful step forward. Each meal brings you closer to becoming proficient at burning a clean, rich, sustained form of energy. Each drop in carbohydrate, each rise in healthy fats, each careful addition of fluids and sodium — all these tweaks align to move you toward a state of metabolic flexibility.

As you progress through the first two weeks of your 30-Day Transformation, you may find your body beginning to respond in remarkable ways. Your energy starts to stabilize, no longer subject to dramatic drops and surges. Your cravings diminish, particularly for sweets and processed carbohydrates. Your mental clarity improves; you find yourself thinking more sharply, focusing more easily, and experiencing a newfound calm in your daily routines. Naturally, this corresponds to a dramatic reduction in the fluctuations of blood glucose and insulin — a key feature of the ketogenic lifestyle — which lets your body produce energy in a smoother, more sustained, and more efficient way.

This state of nutritional ketosis is measurable and trackable. If you wish, you can use urine test strips or a small, simple finger-prick meter to check for the presence of ketones in your urine or blood. Ideally, you will aim for a blood ketone level of 0.5–3.0 mmol/L — a range that signals your body is predominantly using fatty acids and ketones for energy instead of glucose. Although testing is not a necessity for everyone, it can be a helpful tool for those who want hard data on their progress.

During these middle days — roughly days 10–20 — your meal plan will reflect your growing ability to rely on fatty acids for energy. Naturally, you will consume a diet rich in healthy fats — avocado, olive oil, fatty cuts of grass-fed meats, wild-caught oily fish — alongside a small but appropriate amount of high-caliber proteins. Your carbohydrate intake will remain under 50 grams per day, predominantly from non-starchy veggies — asparagus, zucchini, peppers, and a handful of strawberries or raspberries. The result is a plate filled with rich, savory foods that nourish you without overloading your body with glucose.

Activity during this period can gradually become more strenuous if you wish, reflecting your growing metabolic flexibility. Short, higher-intensity sessions — resistance training, sprints, or high-intensity intervals — may be well-tolerance now that your body efficiently converts fatty acids into energy. Nevertheless, it's crucial to listen to your body and avoid overtraining; this is a time of adaptation and healing, not punishment. Your recovery will be faster, your muscles less prone to soreness, and your ability to perform at a high level will slowly return — often surpassing your previous capabilities — once you're fully adapted.

Hydration and electrolyte intake remain key components of this process. Without proper fluids and sodium, you may suffer from muscle cramps, weakness, or a persistent feeling of lethargy — symptoms sometimes called "keto flu." To avoid this, consider adding a pinch of sea salt to your water, consuming a warm bowl of bone broth, or adding avocado and dark green veggies to your plate. These rich sources of sodium, potassium, and magnesium will help maintain proper muscle and nerve function.

Your calendar for this period might reflect this growing flexibility. Your meal plans may allow for greater variety — adding in different cuts of meats, swapping avocado oil for ghee or olive oil, or trying a rich, creamy avocado-coconut soup. Your physical activity may increase in intensity or duration, reflecting your growing ability to produce energy efficiently from your own body's resources.

Your progress will be measurable in numerous ways. The scale may reflect a drop in weight, predominantly from a reduction in water and a gradual thinning of body-fat stores. Your jeans may fit more loosely, your face may appear thinner, and your muscles may become more defined. Importantly, these physical signals often align with subjective signals — a newfound ease in movement, a sustained energy through the day, a dramatic reduction in cravings and "food noise"— the persistent chatter in your mind that previously demanded a carbohydrate fix.

Your health markers, if you were to check them, would reflect this dramatic internal shift. Fasting glucose drops into a healthy range, HDL climbs upward, and triglycerides diminish. Your blood pressure drops, reflecting a reduction in sodium retention and a relaxation of your vasculature. In many cases, people find their metabolic health improving across the board — a phenomenon sometimes called "metabolic renewal"— when they follow this regimen carefully and consistently.

Your mood and mental clarity, meanwhile, become powerful signals of progress. The fluctuations you previously experienced — nervous energy followed by a dramatic slump — diminish, yielding to a steady, calm, clear state of mind. Your ability to concentrate, handle stress, and find peace under pressure grows. Some people find their anxieties ease and their outlook on life become more optimistic — a reflection of deep, metabolic healing in the nervous system and the reduction of neuroinflammation.

Sleep, an often-overlooked component of health, typically improves during this period as well. Your body finds its circadian rhythms more stable, melatonin production increases in a healthy pattern, and deep, restful sleep becomes your new normal. Many people report falling asleep more easily, staying asleep without waking, and feeling profoundly rested upon awakening — a dramatic contrast to the restless nights and poor recovery previously associated with a carbohydrate-heavy diet.

CHAPTER 8 — SETTING YOUR MACROS

Setting your macros is the key that unlocks the true power of a ketogenic lifestyle. It's not a guessing game, and it certainly isn't a restrictive diet; it's a powerful, flexible way of eating that lets you nourish your body in a way it was meant to be fueled. The first step in this transformation is understanding exactly what your body needs in order to produce energy efficiently, lose unwanted body-fat, stabilize your blood sugar, and keep you feeling strong, clear, and vital day after day. It all comes down to a careful balance of macronutrients — fats, proteins, and carbohydrates — tailored to your unique physiology.

Picture your plate as a carefully constructed masterpiece, a perfect blend of rich, creamy avocado, fatty cuts of grass-fed steak or wild-caught fish, a handful of crispy, non-starchy veggies tossed in a generous amount of pure olive oil or rich, pastured butter. The proportions aren't arbitrary; they reflect a deep understanding of human physiology — how your body converts food into energy and performs its countless daily operations.

Your diet should be composed of roughly 70–80% healthy fats. That might seem dramatic at first, especially if you're used to a diet heavy in carbohydrates and low in fats, but there's a powerful logic to this. Fats are a slow-burning, rich energy source — a literal "fuel brick" — that your body can rely on for sustained energy and stability. They produce less metabolic waste, foster less inflammation, and allow your body to produce ketones, a powerful and efficient form of energy that your brain and muscles love. Naturally rich sources of healthy fats — avocado, olive oil, fatty cuts of meat, macadamia nuts — become your primary calorie contributors, making you feel satiated, reducing cravings, and freeing you from the rollercoaster of blood sugar drops.

Protein should account for 15–20% of your calories. It plays a key role in maintaining muscle mass, repair, and recovery, and it assists in numerous metabolic processes — from making hormones and neurochemicals to keeping your immune system strong. But it's a delicate balance. Eating too much protein can undermine ketosis by triggering a process called gluconeogenesis — where excess amino acids are converted into glucose — adding an unwanted glucose stream into your system and blurring your ability to become fully adapted. So while you want enough to maintain muscle and proper body repair, you need to avoid overconsumption. Lean cuts of grass-fed steak, wild-caught fish, pastured chicken thighs, or rich, fatty cuts — combined with a small amount of plant proteins — help you stay within this range.

Your carbohydrate intake should be kept under 10%. Ideally, you will aim for 20–50 grams of total carbohydrates per day — predominantly from non-starchy veggies — to avoid adding a glucose load that will undermine your progress. Naturally, this means avoiding bread, rice, pasta, soda, and sweets — but it certainly doesn't translate to a barren plate.

There are numerous low-carbohydrate foods rich in fiber and nutrients — zucchini, asparagus, broccoli, peppers, avocado — that provide texture, color, and a small amount of carbohydrate without spiking your blood sugar.

How much you need — in total calories and in grams of each macronutrient — depends on a range of factors unique to you. Your activity level, age, gender, goals, and health conditions all influence your requirements. If you're a young, physically-active person trying to lose a small amount of body-fat while preserving muscle, you may need a higher calorie intake and more protein than someone who is sedentary and simply wants to lose weight safely and gradually. An older person, a woman in menopause, or someone with diabetes will have different requirements altogether.

Using a simple formula, you can find your total calorie needs first. Multiply your body weight by a base number — typically 11–13 calories per pound — and then adjust upward or downward based on your activity level and goals. If you're very sedentary, you might multiply by 11; if you're more active, you might use 13. The result is a ballpark number — the total calories you need each day to maintain your current weight — which you can then adjust downward to lose weight or upward if you aim to put on muscle.

Once you have your total calories, applying these percentages is fairly simple. If you need 1,800 calories a day and you know you want 70% from fats, 20% from proteins, and 10% from carbohydrates, you multiply 1,800 by 0.7, 0.20, and 0.10, respectively. That means you'd aim for 1,260 calories from fats, 360 from proteins, and 180 from carbohydrates. Divide these calorie amounts by 9 for fats, 4 for proteins and carbohydrates, and you have your grams. So 1,260 divided by 9 equals 140 grams of healthy fats; 360 divided by 4 equals 90 grams of protein; and 180 divided by 4 equals 45 grams of carbohydrate — which you will predominantly fill with non-starchy veggies.

Using an online macro calculator can streamline this process. There are numerous free resources that allow you to plug in your age, sex, weight, activity level, and goals and quickly generate your tailored macronutrient breakdown. Some will even produce meal plans and grocery lists to match your macronutrient goals. But whether you use a calculator or do it manually, understanding these fundamentals is key. It lets you adjust and fine-tune your diet based on your progress, preferences, and health goals.

Setting your macros accurately is more than just a numbers game; it's a powerful tool for staying in ketosis, for seeing results, and for honoring your body's unique needs. It lets you move forward with confidence and clarity, assured that you're not guessing or following a one-size-fits-all diet, but designing a lifestyle that's tailored to you.

As you become more comfortable dialing in your macronutrient intake, you'll find a remarkable transformation beginning to take place in your body and mind. Your energy levels will stabilize; you'll no longer suffer from the dramatic drops in mood and motivation that come from a carbohydrate-heavy diet. Your cravings will diminish and then fade, freeing you from the temptation of sweets and processed foods. Instead of battling hunger all day, you will find a deep, sustained satiety from rich, nourishing foods. Your body will learn to efficiently utilize its own stored energy — the body-fat you wish to lose — alongside the healthy fats you eat.

This process — the metabolic shift into ketosis — depends directly on staying within your macronutrient ratios. If you suddenly consume more carbohydrate than your body can handle, your glucose will rise, your insulin will follow, and this will undermine your ability to produce ketones and to become fully adapted. That's why we say it's not just about total calories; the macronutrient proportions profoundly affect how your body parses and utilizes energy. It's this careful balance — high in healthy fats, moderate in proteins, and very low in carbohydrates — that lets you become a proficient fat-burner instead of a carbohydrate-burner.

Protein plays a particularly delicate role in this process. Too much, and it converts to glucose; not enough, and you undermine your ability to maintain muscle and repair tissues. That's why we aim for 15–20% of total calories — a range that seems to be "just right" for most people. Naturally, there is some variation; a highly-active person might need more, an elderly person might need less. But this range lets you maximize benefits without adding excess to be turned into glucose.

Healthy fats form the basis of your calories. They provide sustained energy, aid in the absorption of vitamins, help produce and regulate key hormones, and form the structure of your cell membranes. Naturally, choosing the right kind of fats is crucial. Ideally, you will consume predominantly monounsaturated and saturated fats from whole, unprocessed sources — avocado, olive oil, fatty cuts of grass-fed and pastured meats, wild-caught fatty fish — while minimizing the intake of industrial seed oils, hydrogenated fats, and trans-fats. Naturally rich sources of omega-3 fatty acids, such as fatty fish and flaxseed, help to reduce inflammation and promote cardiovascular health.

Your carbohydrate intake should come primarily from non-starchy, low-glycaemic sources — leafy greens, cruciferous veggies, peppers, zucchini — that provide fiber, micronutrients, and antioxidants without adding a large glucose load. Ideally, you will aim for 20–50 grams of total carbohydrate per day, which typically corresponds to under 10% of total calories. Importantly, this comprises total carbohydrate; some people find it helpful to track net carbohydrate instead — total carbohydrate minus fiber — to reflect more accurately the amount of carbohydrate available for energy.

Once you have calibrated these macronutrient proportions to match your calorie intake and goals, meal planning becomes a much more purposeful and rewarding process. It guides you toward choosing foods that align with your goals and away from those that undermine them. It lets you put together a plate that you know will nourish you, keep you satiated, and allow you to progress toward your health goals, whether you want to lose weight, control diabetes, reduce inflammation, or simply feel more energetic and clearer.

Using an online macro calculator is a helpful starting point, but your own experience will be your greatest teacher. As you follow this plan for a few days or weeks, you will start to observe how your body responds — your energy, your hunger signals, your weight, your health markers — and you can fine-tune your intake to match your goals. If you find you're losing muscle or feeling weak, you may need to raise your protein slightly; if you're not losing body-fat, you may need to cut back a bit on total calories or carbohydrate. The key is flexibility and awareness — honoring your body's signals and making small, purposeful adjustments until you find your own "sweet spot."

This iterative process — dialing in your macronutrient intake — is a powerful form of self-discovery. It lets you connect directly with your physiology and learn what makes you flourish. The ketogenic diet isn't a rigid set of rules; it's a framework — a powerful tool — that you customize and fine-tune to match your unique needs. The result is a way of eating that feels effortless and empowering, a lifestyle you can maintain and enjoy for years to come.

CHAPTER 9 — FOODS TO EAT AND FOODS TO AVOID

Walking into a grocery store when you're first starting a ketogenic diet can feel overwhelming. The array of choices — the colorful produce, the countless packages, the rows upon rows of processed foods — can make it hard to know exactly what you should put in your basket and what you should leave on the shelf. But once you learn the principles of ketogenic eating and become proficient at identifying foods that align with those principles, grocery shopping transforms from a confusing experience into a purposeful and empowering one. Your choices become an opportunity to nourish your body, control your health, and move forward on your transformational journey.

Healthy fats form the foundation of your plate on a ketogenic diet. Naturally rich sources of monounsaturated and saturated fats — foods like avocado, olive oil, coconut oil, and fatty cuts of fish — become your main energy providers. There's a deep logic to this. Your body has a remarkable ability to efficiently use fatty acids for energy and produce ketones when carbohydrate intake drops. It's a process we were designed for — a metabolic state we revert to when food is scarce or when we limit carbohydrate intake. The result is a more stable, sustained form of energy, without the dramatic fluctuations in blood sugar and the corresponding drops in energy and cravings.

Avocados are a perfect example of a food rich in healthy monounsaturated fats and fiber — a true superstar in the ketogenic diet. They're creamy, versatile, and filled with nutrients. Whether you slice them into a salad, blend them into a creamy guacamole, or spoon them directly from their skin, avocados provide a rich, satiating texture alongside numerous health benefits. They're a rich source of potassium, a key electrolyte that many people become deficient in when starting ketogenic dieting.

Olive oil — particularly extra-virgin — is another health-conscious choice. It's rich in oleic acid and polyphenols, compounds that help reduce inflammation and protect against chronic disease. Coconut oil, meanwhile, contains medium-chain triglycerides (MCTs), a form of fatty acid that converts directly into ketones and can be a powerful tool during the adaptation phase to help ease the body into ketosis. There's a rich tradition of health practitioners prescribing MCT oil to help people produce ketones more quickly and efficiently.

Protein, meanwhile, plays a crucial role in a ketogenic diet — not in excess, but in appropriate amounts. Your body needs sufficient protein to maintain muscle mass, repair tissues, produce essential hormones and neurochemicals, and keep you feeling strong and satiated. But it's a delicate balance; consuming more than you need can undermine ketosis by triggering a process called gluconeogenesis, where excess amino acids are converted into glucose. That's why choosing rich, whole food sources of proteins — grass-fed beef, chicken thighs, wild-caught fatty fish — makes a huge difference. Naturally fatty cuts of meat, like a well-marbled steak or crispy-skinned chicken thighs, provide a rich blend of proteins and fats in the proportions your body prefers.

Fish, especially fatty varieties like wild-caught salmon, mackerel, or sardines, is a powerful food for a ketogenic lifestyle. It's rich in omega-3 fatty acids, which help combat inflammation and protect against chronic disease, and it provides a complete profile of essential amino acids. Furthermore, these varieties are typically lower in mercury and other toxins, making them a health-conscious choice.

Non-starchy veggies — leafier varieties like spinach, kale, and lettuce; cruciferous veggies like broccoli and cauliflower; colorful options like peppers and zucchini — bring texture, fiber, and nutrients without adding a large carbohydrate load. They help keep you feeling full, aid in digestion, and provide numerous vitamins and antioxidants that you need for overall health and well-being. Naturally rich in fiber, these foods slow the absorption of nutrients, adding a stability to your blood sugar and helping you avoid dramatic fluctuations in energy and mood.

Nuts and seeds can be a wonderful addition in small amounts. They're rich in monounsaturated fats, magnesium, and other micronutrients. Macadamia nuts, almonds, pistachios, flaxseeds, and chia are all viable options, provided you consume them in moderation and account for their carbohydrate content. Naturally, this means you shouldn't eat them by the handful, but adding a small amount to a salad or yogurt can be a great way to boost texture and flavor.

Dairy products can be a convenient and rich addition to a ketogenic diet, provided you choose varieties that are high in fat and low in carbohydrates. Aged hard cheeses, heavy cream, and full-fat yogurt (without added sugars) can be incorporated in reasonable amounts. Naturally, this depends on your tolerance; some people find dairy to be inflammatory or hard to digest and may need to avoid it. Nonetheless, for many, it adds a rich texture and taste to their diet and makes meal planning more enjoyable.

Forbidden foods — the ones you should avoid — follow a clear principle: anything rich in carbohydrates, processed, or filled with hidden sugars. Bread, pasta, rice, potato, soda, and sweets are all off-limits. Naturally, these foods cause dramatic fluctuations in blood sugar and undermine the ability to produce ketones. They promote a state of dependency on glucose instead of a state of metabolic flexibility — a key objective for those following a ketogenic lifestyle.

Most processed and deep-fried foods should be avoided due to hidden carbohydrates and industrial seed oils — which are often rich in omega-6 fatty acids and can promote chronic inflammation. Foods like potato chips, crackers, French fries, and fast food typically combine poor carbohydrate sources with poor-fat sources — a perfect recipe for metabolic dysfunction.

Your main focus should be whole, unprocessed foods — ingredients that you can pronounce, that your great-grandparents would recognize as food, and that come directly from nature. There's a rich simplicity to this approach. It lets you nourish yourself in a way that's true to human physiology — honoring your body's ability to produce energy from a range of sources and to maintain health without the dramatic fluctuations in blood sugar and energy that come from a carbohydrate-heavy diet.

This chapter aims to empower you to make choices with confidence, simplifying your grocery shopping, meal planning, and cooking. The result is a plate filled with rich, satisfying foods — a plate designed to produce health, not disease; energy, not weakness; clarity, not confusion; and a deep, sustained transformation of your body and mind.

As you become more proficient at choosing foods that align with a ketogenic lifestyle, you will find a wonderful synergy developing between what you eat and how you feel. Your body starts to respond positively — energy levels become more stable, mental clarity sharpens, and cravings diminish. Your mood may lift, and you find you can concentrate more effortlessly, perform physical tasks with greater ease, and appreciate food in a deep, purposeful way.

This newfound connection to your diet comes from honoring your physiology. The human body was designed to rely predominantly on fats for energy when carbohydrate intake drops. Naturally, when you cut back on bread, pasta, and soda — those ubiquitous sources of processed carbohydrates — your body signals a metabolic shift. It starts to produce ketones from fatty acids in the liver and to use those ketones in addition to fatty acids directly for energy. Your muscles, your heart, and your brain all become proficient at consuming these compounds. The result is a state of metabolic flexibility — a ability to move effortlessly between different sources of energy — and a dramatic reduction in the rollercoaster effects of a high-carbohydrate diet.

This transition highlights the powerful role food plays in health and disease. The very foods you choose to put into your body can profoundly affect your physiology, your biochemistry, and your future health. It's not about counting calories or following a restrictive regimen; it's about choosing foods that align with your body's natural mechanisms for energy production and healing.

Picture your plate filled with rich cuts of grass-fed steak, crispy-skinned chicken thighs, wild-caught fatty fish, buttery avocado, a handful of almonds or macadamia nuts, a serving of zucchini tossed in olive oil, a small side of creamy cauliflower mash — all rich, savory foods that nourish you from the inside. Each meal becomes an opportunity to provide your body with the building blocks it needs for energy, repair, and renewal.

Your grocery list starts to reflect this transformation. The center aisles filled with processed, packaged foods become less and less relevant to you, and you gravitate toward the perimeter — the produce, the butcher, the seafood counter — where whole, unprocessed ingredients are abundant. Your shopping habits become a form of empowerment; you learn to vote with your dollars for foods that align with health, not disease. The food industry, in turn, starts to respond to this demand by offering more grass-fed, organically raised, and naturally processed products — a ripple effect that benefits not just you but future generations.

This approach to food extends into meal preparation, cooking, and dining itself. The ketogenic lifestyle invites you back into your own kitchen, reconnects you with cooking, and deepens your understanding of ingredients and techniques. Making a creamy avocado salad, a rich steak with a side of buttery zucchini, or a savory omelette filled with veggies and cheddar become more than just a means of nourishment; they become a form of creativity, relaxation, and care — for yourself and for those you love.

Some people find it helpful to meal plan and prep in advance — cooking large batches of food at the start of the week and portioning it into meal-sized containers. That way, when you're busy or pressed for time, you have something ready to eat that supports your goals. Others prefer to cook daily, letting their mood and preferences guide their choices. Whatever your style, the key is choosing ingredients that align with a ketogenic lifestyle — rich in healthy fats, proteins, and non-starchy veggies — and avoiding those that undermine it.

Flavors become more pronounced when you cut back on processed ingredients and added sugars. The natural taste of a perfectly grilled steak, a creamy avocado, or a handful of buttery macadamia nuts brings a deep satisfaction. Herbs, garlic, chili flakes, lemon juice, and other seasonings add character and depth to your dishes without adding unwanted carbohydrates. The result is a rich, savory diet that feels indulgent, not restrictive.

Your body responds by shifting its metabolic machinery toward this new way of eating. Inside your cells, numerous biochemical pathways become more efficient at breaking down fatty acids and ketones for energy. Your mitochondria — the powerhouses of your cells — become more numerous and more robust. Your ability to generate sustained energy without dramatic drops or cravings improves. The result is a lifestyle that feels effortless and empowering, a dramatic contrast to the restrictive, calorie-centric diets you may have tried in the past.

Your health markers reflect these internal changes. Your blood sugar drops and stabilises; your HDL — the protective form of cholesterol — climbs; your LDL particles become large and fluffy instead of small and dense; your triglycerides diminish; your C-reactive protein — a marker of chronic inflammation — drops; and your blood pressure normalises. Your body-fat drops while muscle is preserved. Furthermore, many people find their skin clears, their joints become less painful, their headaches diminish, and their gastrointestinal symptoms resolve.

This is not a coincidence; it's a direct result of choosing foods that align with human physiology. The ketogenic diet reduces the metabolic stress placed on the body by chronically elevated glucose and insulin. It dampens the production of reactive oxygen species and the chronic, low-grade inflammation that underpins many modern disorders. It lets your body resolve health issues from the inside — a powerful form of healing that comes not from a medication or a supplement but from choosing the right food.

As you become more proficient at this lifestyle, you will learn to navigate social situations, dining out, and holidays with confidence and ease. The principles you have mastered — choosing whole, low-carbohydrate foods and honoring your body's signals — will guide you no matter where you find yourself. Whether you're sitting at a restaurant, a friend's dinner party, or a family barbecue, you will know exactly what to select from the menu, what to avoid, and how to stay true to your goals without feeling deprived or isolated.

Your friends and family may become curious. They may ask you what you're doing differently, how you're losing weight, feeling more energetic, or improving your health. Naturally, this opens the door for you to become a guide, a role model, and a source of knowledge for those who wish to follow a similar path. Your transformation then ripples forward, influencing not just your own health but the health of those you care about.

The ketogenic lifestyle is a powerful tool — a way to align your diet with your physiology, your goals, and your health. It transforms not just your body but your relationship with food, your understanding of nourishment, and your ability to care for yourself and your future. The foods you eat become a form of medicine, a medium through which you can heal, grow, and flourish.

CHAPTER 10 — PANTRY STAPLES AND MUST-HAVES

Your ketogenic journey finds its true power in your ability to nourish yourself effortlessly and consistently. The key to making this lifestyle not just a temporary diet but a permanent way of living lies in your preparation — in having a well-stocked, purposeful pantry filled with ingredients that align with your health goals. Inside these doors, you should find not temptation or confusion but a rich array of components that empower you to create delicious, satisfying, and healing food without stress or overwhelm.

Picture your ideal ketogenic kitchen. The shelves are neatly filled with ingredients that form the basis of countless savory, rich, and deeply satisfying meals. At your fingertips are cooking fats that not only taste wonderful but also provide a pure, dense energy to nourish you. Among these, avocado oil stands tall, a neutral-tasting, stable oil perfect for high-heat cooking; ghee, rich in short-chain fatty acids and conjugated linoleic acid, adds a rich, buttery depth to your dishes; and pure coconut oil brings its medium-chain triglycerides, or MCTs, to help produce ketones quickly and efficiently.

Nuts and seeds find a permanent home in your ketogenic kitchen, offering texture, flavor, and a convenient way to add a bit of rich, healthy fats and fiber into your diet. Among them, almonds — whether raw, blanched, or ground into flour — become a versatile base for both sweet and savory creations. Chia and flax seeds, tiny yet powerful, bring a dramatic boost of fiber and omega-3 fatty acids; you can fold them into smoothies, use them to make a low-carbohydrate "pudding"—even employ them as a thickening agent in sauces and gravies.

Your panty should also be a refuge for convenient sources of rich, fatty proteins — canned fatty fish, for example, like sardines and mackerel. Naturally rich in omega-3s and calcium (because you eat the tiny, soft bones), these small cans become a savory, convenient meal when you're short on time. A rich, savory bone broth, meanwhile, made from the slow-simmered knuckles and joints of pastured animals, adds a deep umami base to soups, sauces, and braises — or can be sipped warm from a mug, delivering a rush of nutrients directly to your gut and joints.

Flavors come alive in a ketogenic diet when you learn to appreciate the power of herbs, garlic, turmeric, chili flakes, and other seasonings. Naturally carbohydrate-free or extremely low in carbohydrates, these ingredients allow you to illuminate your plate without adding hidden sugars or starch. Herbs like rosemary, thyme, and basil bring a fresh, aromatic depth; chili flakes add a warming kick; turmeric not only lends color and earthiness but also a powerful anti-inflammatory compound called curcumin. Garlic, diced or pressed, adds its pungent, rich flavor to nearly everything — transforming simple ingredients into something extraordinary.

For those moments when you miss a touch of sweetness — and we all have those from time to time — having a small selection of non-caloric sweeteners on hand can be a powerful tool. Naturally-derived options like stevia or erythritol satisfy that sweet tooth without affecting your blood sugar or kicking you out of ketosis. A few drops of liquid stevia in a creamy dessert, or a small amount of erythritol blended into a batter made from almond or coconut flour, can allow you to enjoy a treat without straying from your path.

Flour alternatives are a key component of a well-prepared ketogenic pantry. Traditional flours made from grains are heavy in carbohydrates and undermine your ability to stay in ketosis, but this is where ingredients like blanched almond flour and finely ground coconut flour come into play. With these, you can bake cookies, bread-like treats, pizza crusts, and more — all while keeping carbohydrate content to a minimum and honoring your body's metabolic preferences.

Your collection should be finished off with a carefully curated array of vinegars, mustards, and sauces — all without added sugars — to add a spark of acidity, a touch of umami, or a rich depth to whatever you're preparing. Apple cider vinegar, for example, brings a tart brightness to salad dressings and marinades. Naturally brewed mustard adds a pungent kick to meats and veggies. Tamari — a gluten-free, lower carbohydrate form of soy sauce — delivers a deep, savory flavor perfect for stir-fries and sauces.

Setting up your ketogenic pantry in this way is more than a matter of practicality; it is a form of empowerment. It means you are no longer at the mercy of temptation or confusion when mealtime rolls around. Instead of staring into the refrigerator and wondering what you can eat, you will find yourself surrounded by ingredients you know, love, and trust

— components that align with your health goals and allow you to create delicious, satisfying food quickly and effortlessly.

This preparedness reduces stress, saves time, and cuts down on impulsive choices. It lets you respond to hunger gracefully, without falling back into old habits. It transforms your diet from something restrictive into something rich and abundant — a way of honoring your body's signals and nourishing it profoundly.

Your well-stocked ketogenic pantry becomes a kind of anchor in your lifestyle — a base from which you can explore, innovate, and enjoy a rich array of food without feeling deprived. Whether you're putting together a quick meal after a hectic day or planning a festive dinner to share with friends, you have everything you need at your fingertips.

The result is a dramatic shift in your relationship with food. Your choices become purposeful and empowering, reflecting not a restrictive regimen but a deep understanding of what your body needs to flourish. The ingredients you keep close at hand become the literal building blocks of your health, your energy, and your future.

As you become more comfortable navigating this lifestyle, you will find your well-equipped ketogenic pantry evolves into a kind of creative workshop — a place where you can pursue health through food in a way that's both indulgent and purposeful. The ingredients you stock become your raw materials for a rich, satisfying diet — a diet designed not just for weight control, but for metabolic healing, sustained energy, and a newfound freedom from cravings.

Picture this: you come home after a hectic day, you're a little tired and a little hungry, and you're not sure what you want to eat. But when you opened your cupboard and fridge, you find a world of possibilities. There are cans of wild-caught sardines and mackerel rich in omega-3s; a bag of chia seeds you can transform into a creamy pudding; jars of rich bone broth you can sip to revive yourself; an assortment of herbs and chili flakes you can use to create a savory meal in minutes. Your past self might have felt stressed or unsure, turning to processed or convenient foods in a moment of weakness — now you have everything you need at your fingertips to nourish yourself quickly and effortlessly.

This is a key psychological shift in following a ketogenic lifestyle. It's not a diet of scarcity; it's a way of abundance — a rich array of foods that empower you to be creative, flexible, and in control. The ingredients you keep in your home reflect your values and your goals. They say: "I care about my health. I care about honoring my body. I care about making choices that align with my future." That is a powerful affirmation — a daily, actionable affirmation — that transforms your relationship with food from a battleground into a sanctuary.

Of course, this kind of transformation is a process. It starts with education — understanding which ingredients align with your goals and which undermine them. But knowledge without preparation is weak; that's where your well-stocked pantry comes into play. It converts knowledge into action. It makes it effortless to follow through on your choices, meal after meal, day after day.

Flour alternatives like blanched almond flour and coconut flour are a perfect example of this. Traditionally, when you went into your kitchen in search of something sweet or a bit indulgent — a muffin, a piece of bread — you were forced into choosing something made from refined flour and filled with carbohydrates. That kind of food quickly converts into glucose, spiking your blood sugar and adding to a cascade of metabolic dysfunction. But now you have a powerful alternative. A handful of ingredients from your ketogenic pantry can become a rich, moist muffin or a crispy loaf of bread — all without adding a rush of glucose into your body.

This ability to transform ordinary ingredients into something extraordinary underscores a key principle of the ketogenic lifestyle: it's not about suffering or going without; it's about honoring your body while honoring your senses and your traditions. The rich taste of a warm loaf made from coconut flour, a handful of herbs, and a few farm-fresh eggs can connect you to a deep, universal feeling of nourishment — without derailing your health goals.

Your collection of vinegars, mustards, and sauces plays a similar role. Naturally carbohydrate-free or very low in carbohydrates, these ingredients allow you to add depth, acidity, and complexity to your dishes without adding hidden sugars or starch. A squeeze of apple cider vinegar can cut through the richness of a fatty meal, adding brightness and balance. A spoonful of mustard can create a creamy, savory sauce for grilled meats or hard-cooked eggs. Tamari can bring a rich umami depth to a vegetable stir-fry or a marinade for steak. All of these ingredients empower you to produce food that feels indulgent, sophisticated, and profoundly satisfying — without straying from your health goals.

Non-caloric sweeteners, meanwhile, are a powerful tool for those moments when you want a treat. A few drops of liquid stevia in your coffee, or a small amount of erythritol blended into a batter made from almonds and coconut, lets you enjoy a rich, sweet flavor without disturbing your metabolic state. Importantly, these sweetening strategies enable you to celebrate, to treat yourself, and to connect with traditions — birthday parties, holiday treats, and festive foods — without feeling deprived or ostracized.

Your well-stocked ketogenic pantry lets you appreciate food for what it is meant to be: nourishment, a medium for creativity, a way to connect with your surroundings and your traditions, and a powerful tool for health and transformation. It signals a deep shift in how you view food and cooking — not as a restrictive regimen, but as a rich and abundant lifestyle — a lifestyle designed to maximize health, happiness, and human potential.

CHAPTER 11 — 100+ EASY LOW-CARB, HIGH-FAT RECIPES

As you step into this chapter, you're not just opening a collection of recipes — you're entering a world of rich, indulgent food that nurtures you from the inside out. Here, you will find more than 100 easy, low-carbohydrate, high-fat recipes, all carefully crafted to align with a ketogenic lifestyle. Each meal you create from these pages is more than a plate of food; it's a tool for transformation, a key to unlocking your health, energy, and happiness. The power of this collection lies in its simplicity and its ability to bring you back into a deep, ancestral way of eating — a way that focuses on whole, rich ingredients that nourish you without adding needless carbohydrates and processed components.

Every recipe you find here has been designed to be low in carbohydrate and rich in healthy fats — precisely what your body needs to become a proficient fat-burner. The result is a diet that feels indulgent and satisfying while guiding you toward your health goals. It's a paradox that many find hard to believe at first: you're encouraged to eat creamy sauces, rich cuts of meat, buttery veggies, crispy cheeses, and even sweet treats — all while losing weight, improving metabolic health, and experiencing a newfound clarity and energy. There's a kind of magic in this transformation. It's not a restrictive diet; it's a rich lifestyle — a lifestyle made delicious.

The recipes you're about to explore are designed to be simple and quick. There's no need to be a trained chef or a health expert to follow them. Whether you're a busy professional, a parent with a hectic schedule, or someone who simply wants to streamline meal preparation, you'll find these recipes doable and adaptable. Some can be made in under 10 minutes, perfect for those nights when you need something fast and nourishing. Others can be prepared in batches and chilled or frozen for future use — a lifesaver when you want to stay on track without spending hours in the kitchen each day.

Flavors range from savory and hearty to sweet and indulgent. There's a rich diversity here that guarantees you'll find something to suit your taste buds and preferences. From crispy-skinned chicken thighs to creamy avocado smoothies, from buttery seafood dishes to rich, decadent desserts made without a gram of sugar, this collection proves you do not have to suffer or miss out when choosing health. Your plate can be filled with food that is rich in texture, deep in flavor, and profoundly satisfying.

Each recipe comes with a breakdown of macronutrients — grams of carbohydrate, protein, and healthy fats — as well as the net carbohydrate content per serving. This lets you track exactly what you're consuming without guessing or calculating manually. If you have specific goals — whether you aim to stay under 20 grams of net carbohydrate per day or you need more protein to match your activity — these nutritional details empower you to make choices that align with your goals. It transforms meal planning from a confusing puzzle into a clear, actionable process.

This collection covers all meal categories — from savory breakfasts that will keep you feeling full all morning, to hearty lunches and rich, satisfying dinner options, to small snacks and treats that allow you to celebrate without straying from your path. Whatever meal you need, whatever mood you're in, there's something here for you. Whether you're a beginner just starting this lifestyle or a veteran chef who wants to keep their plate fresh and exciting, you will find a recipe to match your needs.

As you move through these pages, you will appreciate how flexible and adaptable this diet can be. The ingredients are readily available — you'll find most of them at your grocery store or nearby market — and you will learn how to combine them in countless ways to produce a rich array of meal options. There's no need to rely on specialized products or hard-to-obtain ingredients. The base components — meats, low-starch veggies, healthy fats, and a few key seasonings — come together effortlessly into something extraordinary.

This collection aims not just to help you stay motivated, delighted, and fully committed to your ketogenic journey, but to show you how much abundance is available to you. The ketogenic lifestyle isn't about counting calories or feeling deprived; it's about choosing a path of nourishment, satisfaction, and freedom. It's about honoring your body's ability to heal, transform, and flourish when given the proper nutrients.

Every meal you create from these pages brings you a step closer to your goals — whether those goals are weight-loss, improved energy, mental clarity, or a reversal of health issues. It's a powerful feeling to know you have control over what you eat and how it makes you feel. Your plate becomes a tool for transformation — a form of daily medicine — made all the more enjoyable by rich flavors and indulgent textures.

So let this collection be your guide, your inspiration, and your daily affirmation. Let these recipes become a part of your lifestyle — a lifestyle filled with health, happiness, and abundance. Embrace this rich, savory journey with an open mind and a willing plate. There's a world of delicious possibilities waiting for you, meal by meal, day by day.

As you move forward in this journey, it's worth reflecting on just how much this collection is designed to empower you. Each meal you prepare from these pages is not an isolated act of cooking; it's a small but powerful affirmation — a renewal of your health goals, a deepening of your understanding of food, and a literal reshaping of your future. The ketogenic diet isn't a restrictive regimen; it's a rich, flexible lifestyle that lets you enjoy food to its fullest while honoring your body's physiology.

Picture your mornings beginning with a creamy avocado and smoked salmon omelette — rich in omega-3s, monounsaturated fats, and proteins that keep you satiated and energized. The texture is silky, the flavor indulgent, yet the meal is profoundly nourishing, aligning with your macronutrient goals without a hint of regret. Naturally low in carbohydrate and rich in nutrients, it sets the tone for a day filled with sustained energy and clarity.

As the day evolves and you move toward lunch, you might find yourself turning to a crispy-skinned chicken thigh salad tossed in a creamy ranch made from avocado oil and herbs. The crispy chicken brings a savory satisfaction, while the creamy ranch adds a rich texture — all without adding unwanted carbohydrates. The combination of protein and healthy fats not only signals satiety to your body but also assists in keeping your blood sugar and insulin levels stable, allowing you to avoid those dramatic energy drops and cravings.

Later, when dinner rolls around, you may opt for a buttery grilled steak alongside a pile of garlicky zucchini noodles tossed in a rich Parmesan sauce. Here, you're honoring your body's need for high-fat, low-carbohydrate nourishment while experiencing a meal that feels indulgent and sophisticated. The savory richness of the steak, combined with the creamy texture of the Parmesan-covered zucchini, highlights how ketogenic cooking lets you enjoy food without feeling deprived.

Of course, snacks and treats have their place in this lifestyle as well — a handful of almonds, a piece of dark chocolate rich in antioxidants, or a creamy peanut butter fudge made without adding a drop of sugar. These small indulgences can be powerful allies in staying the course, helping you conquer cravings and avoid feeling deprived.

One of the greatest misconceptions about ketogenic eating is that it's restrictive or boring. The collection of 100+ recipes here shows just the opposite. It reveals a rich, flexible, and profoundly satisfying way of cooking — a way that lets you celebrate food while honoring health. The ingredients you use — from rich cuts of grass-fed beef and pastured chicken, to wild-caught seafood and creamy cheeses — are abundant in flavor and texture. The diet naturally focuses you on whole, unprocessed ingredients — the kind that nourish your body at a deep, cellular level.

This collection also guides you in meal prepping and planning. If you're a busy person — someone with a hectic career, a family to care for, or numerous responsibilities — you will appreciate how many of these recipes can be made in large batches and kept in the fridge or freezer. Soups, chili, and slow-cooker dishes can be made on a Sunday afternoon and portioned out for the rest of the week. Roasting a large cut of meat — a whole chicken, a pork shoulder, or a brisket — lets you enjoy it in a variety of forms, from salads and omelets to creamy stews.

Your ketogenic journey is not about counting every calorie or feeling hungry; it's about choosing foods that nourish you, heal you, and allow you to flourish. It's about honoring your body's ability to produce its own energy — through ketones — when you cut back on carbohydrates and allow healthy fats to become your main metabolic fuel. The result is a dramatic reduction in cravings, a newfound freedom from food obsession, and a deep, sustained energy that permeates all aspects of your life.

This collection is designed to empower you to find your own path within this lifestyle. There's a rich diversity of cuisines — Mexican, Italian, Mediterranean, and more — all adapted to be low in carbohydrate and rich in healthy fats. Whether you love rich curries, savory roasts, or light, fresh salads, you will find something here to suit your preferences.

Furthermore, these recipes celebrate the pure simplicity of whole foods. There's a deep satisfaction in preparing a meal from ingredients you know and trust — a handful of herbs, a piece of grass-fed steak, a handful of avocadoes — and transforming it into something extraordinary. It reconnects you to cooking as a form of nourishment and artistry, a way to care for yourself and your family.

As you progress through this collection, you will learn techniques to maximize flavor while honoring your health goals. That might be adding a rich compound butter to a piece of grilled steak or finishing a creamy soup with a dollop of heavy cream and crispy bacon. It might be swapping out traditional noodles for zucchini or shirataki, or baking a rich, flourless chocolate torte for a special treat.

Your understanding of food will deepen. The collection guides you toward a greater awareness of macronutrient ratios — which foods are rich in healthy fats, which provide a complete and satisfying source of protein, and which are low enough in carbohydrate to align with your goals. It shows you how to combine ingredients in a way that naturally produces a meal rich in all the components your body needs.

This rich understanding lets you move away from rigid meal plans and toward a more intuitive style of cooking and eating. Once you learn which foods align with your goals and how to prepare them, you will find it effortless to create a meal from whatever you have on hand. Your grocery list will become a flexible guide — filled with foods you know you love and can use to nourish yourself in countless combinations.

Your ability to stay motivated, to find satisfaction in your food, and to progress toward your health goals depends largely on having a rich collection of recipes, techniques, and meal plans at your disposal. That's exactly what this chapter aims to provide. It's not a restrictive diet; it's a rich lifestyle — a powerful way of honoring your health, your goals, and your love of food.

CHAPTER 12 — BREAKFAST IDEAS TO KICKSTART YOUR DAY

The first meal of your day sets the tone for everything that follows — your energy, your mood, your cravings, your ability to stay motivated and clearheaded — it all starts from that moment you break your fast in the morning. If you nourish yourself with a rich blend of healthy fats, proteins, and low-carbohydrate ingredients, you're not just "having breakfast"; you're sending a powerful metabolic signal to your body and mind. You're letting your body know it's time to start burning its own fatty stores for energy instead of begging for a rush of glucose. You're honoring your physiology in a deep and fundamental way.

Picture the moment you sit down to a plate filled with creamy avocado and perfectly cooked eggs — the yolks rich and buttery, the whites firm and delicate — alongside crispy, savory bacon or a few thick slices of smoked salmon. The combination of high-fat and low-carbohydrate foods signals your body to produce ketones, an alternative and more efficient energy source. Naturally, this process dampens hunger signals, provides a sustained release of energy, and lets you move through your morning without the dramatic blood sugar fluctuations that a carbohydrate-heavy breakfast typically brings.

Your choices for a ketogenic breakfast are rich and abundant. The classic omelette, for example, is a perfect canvas for creativity. Fold in diced peppers, zucchini, and a handful of cheddar or mozzarella, and you have a savory meal that delivers a perfect blend of nutrients to kickstart your day. The proteins aid in muscle repair and growth, while the healthy fats provide sustained energy and a feeling of deep satisfaction. Chia pudding is another wonderful option — made by soaking chia seeds in coconut milk or heavy cream overnight — yielding a creamy texture rich in omega-3 fatty acids and fiber, without the carbohydrate rush you'd find in traditional yogurt parfaits.

Protein-rich pancakes made from coconut or almond flour are a popular twist on a classic breakfast treat. They allow you to enjoy something indulgent and comforting while honoring your ketogenic lifestyle. Served with a dollop of whipped cream or a few strawberries, these pancakes are rich in flavor and texture, yet low in carbohydrate and high in healthy fats — perfect for a weekend treat or a special breakfast.

Bacon, a quintessential savory food, plays a key role in many ketogenic breakfasts. Naturally rich in healthy fats and proteins, it delivers a deep, satisfying flavor that pairs well with nearly anything. Combine crispy bacon with creamy avocado, a handful of strawberries, or a pile of buttery scrambled eggs, and you have a meal that is as indulgent as it is nourishing.

For a convenient grab-and-go option, smoothies made from avocado, strawberries, and full-fat coconut milk provide a creamy, rich meal that you can sip on your way to work or after a morning workout. The avocado lends a silky texture and a nice dose of monounsaturated fats, while strawberries add a touch of natural sweetness without overloading you with carbohydrates. Coconut milk brings a rich, tropical flavor and medium-chain triglycerides, which are easily convertible into energy by your body.

Some people find a simple "Bulletproof Coffee"— a blend of strong coffee, grass-fed butter, and MCT oil — is a perfect way to start their day. The result is a rich, creamy beverage that provides sustained energy and mental clarity without the jitters or energy drops associated with a carbohydrate-rich breakfast. MCT oil converts quickly into ketones and provides a convenient, fast-acting energy boost — perfect for busy mornings when you need to be sharp and productive.

For those who prefer savory and hearty breakfasts, frittatas and quiches are a wonderful meal option. They can be filled with a range of ingredients — diced peppers, onions, diced ham, sausage, or creamy cheeses — all blended together with rich, farm-fresh eggs. Frittatas and quiches can be made in advance and cut into convenient single-serving sizes, perfect for meal prepping and staying on track all week long.

This chapter includes more than 20 recipes — a rich and satisfying collection designed to suit all preferences and schedules. Whether you want something sweet or savory, grab-and-go or a sit-down meal, you're going to find something here that fits effortlessly into your ketogenic lifestyle. Each recipe is crafted to be rich in healthy fats, complete proteins, and low in carbohydrate — honoring the macronutrient ratios that allow your body to stay in a state of nutritional ketosis. Your mornings will become a powerful launchpad for a successful day — a day filled with sustained energy, mental clarity, and a deep, rich satisfaction in the food you eat.

As you move forward on your ketogenic journey, you'll find that breakfast evolves from a rushed, hectic meal into a rich opportunity for nourishment and stability. It becomes something you look forward to — a moment to appreciate food in its pure form and to align your choices with your goals for health, energy, and longevity. The key is honoring both simplicity and creativity, making sure you have a repertoire of recipes that match your mood, your schedule, and your preferences.

Some mornings you may want something rich and indulgent, a plate that feels more like a weekend treat — perhaps creamy avocado blended into a savory omelette alongside crispy, thick-cut bacon. Other mornings you might prefer something light, quick, and convenient — a chia pudding you made the night before or a creamy avocado-coconut milk shake blended in minutes. Whatever you choose, you're honoring your body's ability to become a proficient fat-burner.

The possibilities for ketogenic breakfasts are nearly endless, and you're not limited to just the classics. Naturally sweet ingredients — strawberries, raspberries, blackberries — can be incorporated in small amounts to add a fresh, tart flavor. Herbs and spices — chili flakes, dill, turmeric, and paprika — can bring depth and warmth to your dishes. Cheeses — from creamy brie to cheddar to mozzarella — add richness and texture.

Picture a plate of buttery zucchini pancakes made with Parmesan and herbs — crispy on the outside, tender on the inside — alongside a few thick rashers of crispy prosciutto. The savory flavor combines with the rich texture to create a meal that feels indulgent, yet it's entirely compliant with your ketogenic lifestyle. Or consider a creamy cottage cheese bowl tossed with diced strawberries and a handful of chia seeds — a perfect blend of texture, flavor, and nutrients.

Meanwhile, your ability to stay in a state of ketosis during the day depends on making choices at breakfast that align with your macronutrient goals. Naturally, you aim for a meal rich in healthy fats and proteins, with carbohydrate kept to a minimum. Ideally, you're consuming no more than 5–10 grams of net carbohydrate at breakfast — this small amount can come from low-starchy veggies, a handful of strawberries, or a bit of avocado — enough to add texture and flavor without interfering with your ability to produce ketones.

Protein is an essential piece of this puzzle, not only for retaining muscle mass and repair but also for adding satiety and staying power. Foods like eggs, smoked fish, or grass-fed ground beef all provide complete proteins alongside desirable fatty acids. The combination signals your body to release the satiety signals you need to stay feeling full and focused all morning, without experiencing dramatic drops in energy or cravings for sweets.

Healthy fats — from avocado, olive oil, coconut oil, or fatty cuts of meat — are your main energy source in the ketogenic diet. They slow the release of food from your stomach, yielding a sustained flow of energy and keeping you feeling fueled for hours. Furthermore, when you eat a meal rich in healthy fats first thing in the day, you're teaching your body to rely less on glucose and more on fatty acids and ketones.

It's a powerful metabolic shift — a key to unlocking sustained energy and freedom from fluctuations in blood sugar.

Some people find adding medium-chain triglycerides, or MCT oil, to their breakfast — whether in their coffee or smoothies — can help accelerate this process. MCTs are a unique form of fatty acid that converts quickly into ketones, providing an instant and sustained energy boost without adding a large amount of calories or putting stress on the digestive system. If you're new to ketogenic eating, adding a small amount — say, a teaspoon — to your coffee in the morning can be a gentle way to ease into this lifestyle.

The key is designing a breakfast that fits your goals, preferences, and lifestyle — a meal you look forward to and that supports you physically and mentally for hours afterwards. Whether you're a busy professional who needs something fast, a health-conscious parent who wants a family-friendly meal, or an athlete looking to maximize performance, there are countless ketogenic breakfast options to suit your needs.

For meal prepping, consider making a large frittata filled with veggies and meats, then cutting it into segments to grab and eat all week. Chia puddings can be prepared in jars the night before and stored in the fridge, ready to grab in the morning alongside a hardboiled egg or a few avocado slices. Cloud bread — a low carbohydrate, high-fat bread substitute made from eggs and cream cheese — is another versatile base for a savory breakfast sandwich with avocado, tomato, and crispy bacon.

As you become more proficient in this lifestyle, you'll find you naturally gravitate toward foods that nourish you and align with your goals. Your taste preferences will adapt; the cravings for sweet, carbohydrate-rich foods diminish, and your body starts to appreciate rich, savory flavors and creamy textures instead.

CHAPTER 13 — LUNCH FAVORITES TO KEEP YOU SATISFIED

When we talk about staying on track with a ketogenic lifestyle, the middle of the day — when the temptation to grab something convenient or filled with hidden carbohydrates is at its highest — can be a delicate moment. Your choices at lunch profoundly affect your energy, your mood, and your ability to maintain a state of nutritional ketosis well into the afternoon and evening. That's why it's so crucial to have a rich array of hearty, low-carbohydrate meal options that not only nourish you physically but also satisfy you mentally and emotionally. A well-planned, delicious lunch signals to your body and your mind that you're honoring your health goals without feeling deprived or restrictive.

Picture a plate filled with a perfectly grilled, grass-fed burger patty — rich in flavor and texture — resting on a leaf of crispy lettuce instead of a traditional bun. The burger is adorned with creamy avocado, a slice of tomato, crispy pickle, and a dollop of rich, savory mayonnaise. Each component adds its own depth of flavor and texture, transforming something that might normally be a simple fast-food meal into a sophisticated, health-supportive plate. The avocado brings a rich, buttery texture alongside monounsaturated fats that help keep you feeling full. The tomato adds a slight acidity to cut through the richness, while the crispy pickle delivers a satisfying crunch. Altogether, it's a meal that feels indulgent yet it's perfectly aligned with your ketogenic goals.

Protein-rich salads are another wonderful way to maximize both nutrients and satisfaction at lunch. Instead of a plate filled with uninspiring iceberg lettuce, a well-composable salad might start with a base of peppery arugula or rich, dark baby kale. To this, you can add diced grilled chicken thighs, steak strips, or a handful of flaked tuna tossed in a creamy, high-fat dressing made from avocado oil or ranch. Sprinkle in a few olives, diced cucumber, or a handful of strawberries for texture and a small hint of natural sweetness. The result is a meal rich in nutrients, full of texture, and profoundly satisfying — exactly what you need to carry you through the rest of your day without energy drops or cravings.

For those who appreciate a warm bowl of something savory, a rich bone broth soup filled with low-starchy veggies and diced meats can be profoundly comforting. A base made from slow-cooking chicken or beef knuckles results in a broth rich in collagen, amino acids, and mineral content — perfect for strengthening joints and improving gut health. Into this you can add diced zucchini, chopped kale, and small cubes of fatty brisket or chicken thighs. Seasoned to taste with herbs, garlic, and chili flakes, this kind of soup is a perfect meal to sip from a mug or spoon from a bowl — warming you from the inside and delivering a deep, sustained energy.

Noodle lovers need not miss their favorite foods on a ketogenic diet. Zucchini noodles — or "zoodles"— tossed in a creamy alfredo sauce made from heavy cream, Parmesan, and garlic, and then finished with crispy diced pancetta or grilled chicken, makes for a rich and satisfying bowl of "pasta" without all the carbohydrates. The zucchini retains just enough texture to mimic the al dente bite of traditional noodles, while the creamy sauce delivers a rich, indulgent flavor. It's a perfect way to cut back on carbohydrate without losing the feeling of indulgence you associate with your favorite foods.

Another clever option for staying within your carbohydrate goals at lunch is swapping a tortilla for a leaf of lettuce. Large lettuce leaves — from varieties like iceberg or Romaine — can be filled with seasoned ground beef, shredded chicken, diced avocado, salsa, and a dollop of sour cream to create a taco-like experience without the excess carbohydrate of a traditional tortilla. The crispy leaf adds texture and a fresh flavor that highlights all the rich components of the filling. It's a meal that feels fun and indulgent while honoring your health goals.

Slow-cooker and meal-prep friendly options are especially helpful for busy schedules. Anything from a savory chili made without the traditional kidney beans, to a creamy chicken casserole rich in cheese and herbs, can be made in large batches over the weekend and then divided into convenient, grab-and-go containers for the week. Naturally, this cuts back on temptation, prevents waste, and makes sure you always have a satisfying meal within reach. There's a deep peace of mind that comes from opening your refrigerator to find a collection of ready-to-eat, ketogenic-friendly dishes — a true key to staying compliant and feeling supported in your lifestyle.

Leftovers from dinner can become the basis for a wonderful and hearty lunch the following day. A piece of grilled steak, for example, can be diced and tossed into a salad alongside diced cucumber, avocado, hardboiled eggs, and a creamy ranch dressing. Roasted chicken thighs can be shredded and made into a rich chicken salad with a handful of chopped almonds and diced celery. It's a wonderful opportunity to cut back on waste, maximize your grocery budget, and streamline your meal planning.

This chapter contains more than 20 recipes designed to keep your midday meal exciting, satisfying, and profoundly nourishing. Each meal underscores a key principle of the ketogenic lifestyle: we are not deprived; we are choosing rich, whole, savory foods that align with our health goals and leave us feeling energized and well-fueled all afternoon long. Your lunches will become something you look forward to, not a rushed, uninspiring grab-and-go. They will reflect your newfound understanding of food as a powerful tool — not just calories in and calories out — but a means to transform your health from the inside.

As you move forward with your ketogenic journey, allow these meal ideas to become a rich part of your daily rhythm. Take time to appreciate their texture, their flavor, and their ability to nourish you profoundly. The feeling of sustained energy and clarity you experience in the afternoon is a direct result of honoring your body's true needs. It's a dramatic contrast from the energy crashes and cravings that follow a carbohydrate-heavy meal. The ability to move through your day feeling strong, clear, and motivated is a powerful affirmation — a confirmation that you're on the right path.

Your lunches are not a sacrifice; they are a rich opportunity. Each meal is a chance to nourish yourself at a deep level, honoring both your health goals and your taste buds. Whatever you choose — a savory salad, a creamy soup, a plate of zucchini noodles, a lettuce-wrap taco, or a hearty slow-cooker meal — you are not missing a thing. Instead, you're embracing a lifestyle filled with flavor, satisfaction, and a deep, sustained energy that will carry you forward into whatever your day holds. Your lunch, far from being an afterthought, is a key component of your success — a moment to appreciate, nourish, and empower yourself with food.

Your ketogenic lunch is more than just a meal; it's a powerful tool for transformation — a key piece in the puzzle of sustained health and well-being. It's a moment in your day when you are choosing nourishment over temptation, choosing energy over weakness, choosing clarity over fog. Each rich, savory plate you prepare, whether it's a crispy lettuce-wrap filled with ground beef and diced avocado, a creamy zucchini noodle alfredo tossed with diced chicken, or a hearty chili made without the traditional kidney beans, signals a deep honoring of your goals. It reflects a maturity, a discipline, and a deep understanding that food is not your adversary — it's your greatest ally in this journey.

Your ability to create satisfying, ketogenic-friendly lunches lets you break free from a reactive way of eating — a pattern dictated by cravings, poor choices, and scarcity — and move into a lifestyle defined by abundance, satisfaction, and control. The rich fatty cuts of meat, the creamy sauces, the crispy veggies, all serve you in a way that a simple carbohydrate-heavy meal never could. Instead of a dramatic rise and fall in blood sugar, you experience a slow, sustained release of energy, keeping you clear, motivated, and productive through your afternoon hours.

Your choices at lunch ripple forward into the rest of your day. If you nourish yourself properly at midday, you're less likely to suffer from an energy slump at 3 p.m., less prone to cravings in the evening, and more able to make good choices at dinner. The result is a cascade of healthy decisions — a kind of upward spiral — all stemming from honoring your body's true needs. It's a powerful form of momentum. Success feeds upon itself.

Furthermore, choosing rich, whole foods at lunch lets you maximize the health benefits you're experiencing on a ketogenic diet. Your body, freed from the constant fluctuations in blood sugar and the pressure of elevated insulin, can turn its attention toward repair, renewal, and deep healing. Your cells become more proficient at using fatty acids and ketones for energy; your mitochondria become more robust; your body reduces its production of reactive oxygen species; and chronic, low-grade inflammation starts to diminish. All this adds up to a dramatic improvement in health — not just in your physical appearance and energy levels, but in your susceptibility to disease and your ability to age gracefully.

Your ketogenic lunch choices reflect a deep understanding of this process. The rich, fatty cuts of steak or chicken you serve alongside a creamy coleslaw made with a high-fat mayonnaise, or the savory soup you sip made from bone broth and green veggies, all provide the components your body needs to heal, grow, and flourish. Naturally rich in micronutrients, essential fatty acids, and high-digestibility proteins, these foods help to stabilize your mood, cut cravings, and resolve many health issues stemming from poor diet and lifestyle.

As you move forward in your ketogenic journey, you will find that your taste preferences evolve alongside your physiology. The sweet, processed foods that once seemed hard to resist will lose their appeal, while rich, savory, whole foods become deeply satisfying. Your ability to appreciate the subtleties of a creamy avocado, a perfectly grilled piece of steak, or a crispy leaf of lettuce filled with savory ground beef will grow. Your taste buds will become more sensitive to natural flavors, and you will find yourself less and less interested in the overly sweet and overly processed foods that were once a daily temptation.

This transformation — this renewal — starts with choices made at lunch. It starts with honoring your body's signals instead of ignoring them; choosing foods that heal instead of harm; designing a meal plan that supports your goals instead of derailing them. It starts with understanding that food is not simply calories; it's information. It signals your body to either store or release, heal or break down, flourish or struggle. Your plate, in many ways, is a powerful form of communication with your physiology.

So celebrate this moment in your day. Celebrate your ability to nourish yourself in a way that is rich, satisfying, and profoundly health-promoting. Take time to appreciate the meal you're about to eat — to taste it, to enjoy it, and to reflect on the progress you're making. Each ketogenic lunch is a small triumph, a step forward in your health journey.

Your path is not about punishment or deprivation; it's about choosing a lifestyle that lets you become the fullest, healthiest, most energetic person you can be. Your plate is your tool; your choices are your power; and your future is a direct reflection of the choices you make today. So, as you move forward, meal by meal, you are not battling temptation — you are honoring your body and your goals, honoring a future filled with health, happiness, and abundance.

Your ketogenic journey is a rich and rewarding path. At the center of it all is the food you put on your plate — food that sustains, repairs, energises, and transforms you. So let your lunches be a daily affirmation of your goals. Let each meal reflect your knowledge, discipline, and hope for a thriving future. With every rich, satisfying plate, you are choosing health over disease, clarity over confusion, and renewal over deterioration.

Your future starts now — and it starts with your next meal.

CHAPTER 14 — DINNER DELIGHTS TO FINISH STRONG

As the day draws to a close and you reflect on all you have accomplished, dinner becomes more than just another meal — it's a moment of nourishment, a rich opportunity to celebrate the progress you're making and to fortify your body for restful recovery. Your dinner plate is a canvas upon which you can blend indulgence, health, simplicity, and deep satisfaction. It's a time to appreciate all you have done for yourself that day and a chance to close it strong — honoring both your goals and your taste buds.

Picture your plate filled with hearty cuts of steak — rich, fatty, and tender — a perfect centerpiece for a ketogenic meal. The texture melts in your mouth, delivering not just pure satisfaction, but a rich array of nutrients that aid in muscle repair and recovery. Naturally fatty cuts like a well-marbled ribeye or a thick cut of brisket help keep you satiated and provide a sustained release of energy. Complement this with a side of buttery, non-starchy veggies tossed in aromatic herbs — zucchini, asparagus, or green beans — adding texture, color, and a fresh note to balance the rich main course.

Your dinner might take a more homely form in a casserole — a rich blend of cauliflower, ground beef, cheeses, and savory herbs — that feels indulgent without adding carbohydrate load. The creamy texture and hearty components make it a perfect meal for busy nights when you want something warm, comforting, and effortless. It's food that nurtures you from the inside, strengthening you and putting you in a state of deep nourishment. The slow-cooker chili made with diced beef or chicken thighs, peppers, diced tomatoes, and rich broth develops its deep, savory flavor over hours — a perfect solution for a hectic day when you want dinner ready and waiting when you come home.

One-sheet pan recipes cut back on cleanup while delivering robust flavor. Picture a whole chicken thigh tossed in herbs and garlic alongside zucchini, peppers, or brussels sprouts — all crispy and savory by the time they come out of the oven, letting you enjoy a rich meal without messy dishes afterwards. The simplicity of these methods highlights a key principle of ketogenic cooking: you can maximize taste and nourishment without adding needless complexity.

Your dinner plate should reflect a perfect balance — a rich, fatty main alongside a small serving of colorful, low-carbohydrate veggies — yielding a meal that's satisfying without weighing you down. Ideally, this combination signals to your body that it's time to rest, repair, and prepare for a restful, recovery-oriented sleep.

This chapter contains more than 20 meal ideas designed to keep dinner from feeling restrictive or boring. There are Mexican-inspired dishes — chili-lime grilled steak, fajita-style chicken thighs — alongside Italian delights — creamy

Parmesan chicken and zucchini noodles — and Mediterranean classics — grilled lamb chops with olives and herbs — all tailored to a low-carbohydrate lifestyle. Each meal brings its own rich array of flavors and nutrients, reflecting cuisines from all over the world while honoring ketogenic principles.

Your evening meal plays a powerful role in your health journey. It signals to your body that it's time to transition from the active, energetic day into a restful, repair-focused night. The combination of proteins, healthy fats, and low-starchy veggies assists in stabilizing blood sugar, reducing cravings, and preparing you for deep, restful sleep — all crucial components for recovery and renewal. The rich, savory components help you feel full and content, reducing temptation to snack late into the evening.

Your dinner plate is more than just food; it's a tool — a powerful means of honoring your health, your goals, and your future. It's a way to celebrate progress made and a form of deep nourishment for all the systems that keep you thriving.

As you move forward on your ketogenic journey, let dinner be a rich, satisfying affirmation of all you're achieving. Let it be a moment to appreciate the progress you're making and to nourish yourself profoundly in a way that sets you up for future success. Your choices at dinner ripple forward, influencing your rest, recovery, and readiness for the day to come. By choosing rich, indulgent, health-promoting foods, you're honoring both your body and your goals.

So gather your ingredients, prepare your meal, and sit down to appreciate it fully. Let each savory bite connect you to a future filled with health, energy, and confidence — a future you're creating meal by meal, plate by plate.

As you progress further into your ketogenic lifestyle, dinner evolves from a simple meal into a powerful opportunity — a moment where you bring together everything you've learned about low carbohydrate cooking, rich sources of healthy fats, and the importance of high-caliber proteins — to nourish your body at a deep level. It's a time when you can celebrate not just the food itself, but the progress you're making, the discipline you're honoring, and the future you're investing in with each careful choice.

Your dinner plate becomes a reflection of your understanding — a rich blend of savory ingredients that align with your goals and reflect your newfound confidence in choosing what's best for you. Whether you're serving a slow-cooked pot roast, a creamy chicken casserole, or a crispy-skinned piece of fatty fish alongside a medley of low-starchy veggies tossed in herbs and rich butter, you're honoring both your health and your happiness. It's a meal designed not for punishment or scarcity, but for abundance — for a rich experience that feeds you physically and emotionally.

Picture a perfectly seared piece of steak alongside buttery asparagus, or a rich chili made without a single bean but instead filled with savory ground beef, diced peppers, diced tomato, and a blend of warming chili powders. The first bite is pure satisfaction — a rich blend of texture and flavor — proving that you can eat profoundly well while honoring your health goals. Each meal you prepare at dinner underscores a powerful reality: you're not missing out; you're choosing differently, choosing smarter, choosing to nourish yourself from the inside.

Slow-cooking methods allow tough cuts of meat to become tender, yielding rich, savory dishes without adding carbohydrates. Casseroles made from riced cauliflower, ground beef, and cheeses become creamy and indulgent, a perfect marriage of texture and taste. Grilled fatty fish, rich in omega-3s, alongside a creamy dill sauce or a wedge of lemon, brings a fresh, light note to a plate predominantly filled with savory components. Roasting chicken thighs to crispy perfection lets their rich skin become a delivery vehicle for all the rich flavors you love — without adding needless carbohydrates.

Your dinner choices reflect a powerful understanding that food is not your adversary; it's your greatest ally. The ketogenic diet invites you to appreciate food in a new light — honoring its ability to nourish, heal, and empower you. Each meal you serve yourself underscores your progress and affirms your future. It's a form of deep care — for your body, for your health, for your goals.

Flavors from all cuisines find a place at your dinner table — Mexican, Italian, Mediterranean, and more — but all are united by their rich sources of healthy fats and proteins, alongside a careful selection of low-starchy veggies. Fajita-style steak tossed with peppers and a dollop of guacamole brings a festive note to a Wednesday dinner, while creamy chicken thighs in a rich Parmesan sauce transforms a hectic day into a moment of indulgence and relaxation. Roasted lamb chops with herbs and olives celebrate the rich traditions of Mediterranean cooking while honoring your carbohydrate limits. The result is a dining experience that feels abundant, sophisticated, and deeply satisfying.

Your dinner plate is a powerful symbol of renewal — a daily opportunity to nourish your body, reflect on your progress, and celebrate a future filled with health and energy. The rich, savory ingredients you select reflect your understanding of how to align food choices with goals, transforming a meal into a tool for transformation.

As you move forward, you'll find yourself growing more proficient in choosing ingredients, designing menus, and honoring your health without feeling deprived or restrictive. The rich diversity of low-carbohydrate meal options means you will never be bored, never feel that you're missing something, and always appreciate the deep satisfaction that comes from honoring your body's true needs.

Your dinner plate is not a place of scarcity — it's a place of abundance, transformation, and renewal. It's a powerful, daily affirmation that you're choosing health, choosing energy, choosing a future filled with confidence and well-being. Each meal you serve yourself brings you closer to the person you want to become — a person who is strong, vital, and fully alive.

So appreciate each dinner you prepare. Take a moment to reflect on how far you've come and how much further you're going. Let these rich, savory foods nourish you, heal you, and empower you to move forward with confidence and resolve. Your dinner isn't just another meal — it's a key piece of your transformation.

CHAPTER 15 — SNACKS, SIDES, AND APPETIZERS

As you journey forward on your ketogenic lifestyle, you will find that staying the course is not about pure discipline, but about making sure you always have something rich, savory, and satisfying within reach. It's about honoring your body's signals and choosing foods that nourish you, keep you feeling full, and align with your goals — without feeling deprived. Small plate ideas, in the form of snacks, sides, and appetizers, become powerful allies in this process. They conquer cravings gracefully, adding texture, depth, and a wonderful range of flavors to your daily menu.

Healthy snacking on a ketogenic diet can sometimes seem challenging in a world filled with carbohydrate-laden chips, cookies, and candy. But this chapter shows you how easy it is to find indulgences that align with your lifestyle — without kicking you out of ketosis. Instead of gravitating toward processed products, you'll learn to appreciate rich, whole foods that naturally satisfy you. A handful of almonds, a few olives, or a creamy avocado dip can become a convenient grab-and-go option when you need something to keep you fueled and content.

Nuts are a perfect match for this lifestyle — rich in healthy fats, a small handful of almonds, macadamias, or pistachios can be a lifesaver when you're on the move. Pair these with brine-cured olives for a sophisticated, savory combination that feels indulgent but is completely in harmony with your carbohydrate goals. At home, you can prepare creamy avocado dip — a simple blend of avocado, garlic, lemon juice, and herbs — to serve with crispy zucchini chips or raw veggies. It's a rich, velvety dip that lets you enjoy texture and flavor without adding unwanted carbohydrates.

Your ketogenic journey should be filled with small pleasures — foods you love that nourish you at the same time. Deviled eggs are a perfect example. Rich in healthy fats from the yolks and a touch of creamy mayonnaise, tossed with a bit of paprika or herbs, these little treats are a wonderful grab-and-go option or a sophisticated addition to a dinner party plate. The crispy zucchini chips you bake at home, tossed in Parmesan and herbs and then roasted to crispy perfection, serve a similar role — a vehicle for texture and indulgence without straying from your goals.

For a more substantial bite, low carbohydrate meatballs made from ground beef or a mixture of meats can be a perfect small plate, whether you serve them on their own or alongside a creamy dipping sauce made from yogurt or ranch. Bacon-wrapped veggies, whether it's asparagus, peppers, or zucchini, add a rich, savory layer of texture and flavor. The crispy, salty exterior highlights the sweet, tender interior — a perfect blend that feels indulgent and festive.

Sides can be a powerful way to make your main course more satisfying while adding a range of nutrients and texture to your plate. Instead of a heavy potato mash, a creamy cauliflower mash made with heavy cream and butter brings all the rich texture you love without adding excess carbohydrate. Zucchini fritters — crispy on the outside and soft on the inside — serve a similar purpose, adding a wonderful texture alongside your main meal.

Your ketogenic lifestyle should be a rich and enjoyable experience — not a restrictive or barren diet. Small plate recipes allow you to control hunger, adding texture, flavor, and indulgence in a way that supports your health goals. Some can be made in minutes — a handful of olives, a few deviled eggs, a creamy dip — while others, like zucchini fritters or crispy zucchini chips, can be meal-prepped in large batches and kept handy in the fridge.

This collection comprises over 20 side, snack, and appetizer ideas, offering you a rich repertoire to draw from. Whether you're entertaining guests, looking for something to fill you up between meals, or adding a bit of indulgence to your plate, these small plate options will keep you excited about your diet. Your ketogenic lifestyle should be a rich, savory journey — filled with texture, flavor, and the deep satisfaction that comes from honoring your health goals without feeling deprived.

As you move forward, you'll find that having these small plate ideas at your disposal makes all the difference. Your cravings diminish, temptation finds no foothold, and you realize you can enjoy food just as much — if not more — on this lifestyle. So keep these recipes close, meal-prep a few in advance, and allow these rich, savory bites to carry you forward on your path to health, transformation, and renewal. Your ketogenic journey is not about sacrifice; it's about choosing foods that nourish, satisfy, and empower you in every moment.

As you become more comfortable in your ketogenic lifestyle, these small plate ideas will become your greatest tool for staying on track, adding variety, texture, and deep satisfaction to your daily diet. They act as a kind of culinary anchor — something you can rely on when you need a quick meal, a rich side to round out your plate, or simply a small indulgence to keep you feeling rewarded and motivated. The key is having a repertoire you love — a collection of recipes you know by heart, ingredients you always have on hand, and techniques you can execute without stress — so you're never stranded without a delicious, ketogenic-friendly option.

For example, you might find that crispy zucchini chips become your go-to when you want something to crunch on in the evening, swapping potato chips for a rich, savory alternative that's entirely in harmony with your diet. You might learn to appreciate a creamy avocado dip alongside a plate of raw veggies — adding texture and a rich, buttery flavor — or you may discover that a handful of macadamia nuts, tossed in a little chili and rosemary, provides just enough indulgence to satisfy a snack attack without derailing your progress.

Bacon-wrapped veggies, meanwhile, bring a sophisticated twist to your side dishes. The crispy, savory exterior highlights the natural softness and flavor of whatever is within — asparagus, green beans, or zucchini — adding a rich texture that makes a simple vegetable feel indulgent and festive. It's a perfect way to bring a bit of indulgence to your plate without adding needless carbohydrates.

Your small plate repertoire lets you celebrate food in all its forms — rich, creamy, crispy, savory — while honoring your health goals. The key is choosing ingredients that align with your macronutrient ratios — predominantly healthy fats, a small amount of protein, and very few carbohydrates — and putting them together in a way that feels indulgent and satisfying.

Some of these small plate ideas will become your fallback when you're busy and need something quick — a handful of olives, a hardboiled, deviled, or pickled egg, a few crispy zucchini chips — while others may become your centerpieces for entertaining guests or adding a bit of indulgence to a weekend meal. The rich, buttery texture of avocado, the crispy softness of a zucchini fritter, or the creamy richness of a cauliflower mash all bring something special to your plate, making this diet not just a tool for health, but a rich and pleasurable way of eating.

As you progress in your ketogenic lifestyle, you will find your confidence growing alongside your creativity in the kitchen. Small plate cooking lets you appreciate ingredients in their pure form — rich, simple, and satisfying — and lets you control exactly what you put into your body. There are no hidden starches or unwanted preservatives; everything you serve is made from whole, recognizable ingredients.

This approach lets you appreciate food not just for its ability to nourish you, but for its ability to bring you happiness and contentment. The rich texture of a creamy avocado, the savory flavor of crispy bacon, the indulgence of a creamy dip — these all become allies in your health journey, making the path forward feel less restrictive and more abundant.

Your small plate collection lets you customize your diet day by day, choosing a rich side or a savory snack that fits exactly into your lifestyle. Whether you need something quick and convenient or something a bit more sophisticated for a dinner party, you have a range of options at your fingertips. The result is a ketogenic lifestyle that feels rich, indulgent, and satisfying — not restrictive — a way of eating that you can sustain for years to come.

Ultimately, this chapter underscores a key principle of the ketogenic diet: it's not about sacrifice; it's about choosing foods that nourish you profoundly while honoring your love for rich, savory flavors. Small plate cooking lets you do exactly that — transforming ordinary ingredients into extraordinary dishes — and making sure you stay motivated, supported, and delighted on your health journey. Whatever your preferences or lifestyle, these small plate ideas will become a powerful tool for staying on track, feeling satisfied, and truly thriving on a ketogenic diet.

CHAPTER 16 — KETO DESSERTS

It's a wonderful feeling when you realize that a lifestyle change doesn't have to be a sentence to a barren, treat-free future. The ketogenic diet, rich in healthy fats and profoundly low in carbohydrates, isn't about punishment; it's about making choices that nourish you from the inside while honoring those moments when you want a little indulgence, a creamy texture, a rich flavor, or a sweet taste on your tongue. That's where this chapter comes in. Here we celebrate the rich world of ketogenic desserts — treats crafted to align with your goals without derailing your progress — proving you can satisfy your sweet tooth without a dramatic rise in blood sugar or a return to carbohydrate dependency.

Picture this: a smooth, rich chocolate mousse made from avocado and dark chocolate, yielding a creamy texture and deep flavor without adding a heavy carbohydrate load. The avocado provides not only a wonderful mouthfeel but also a rich source of monounsaturated fats and fiber — a perfect match for your ketogenic lifestyle. Sweetening it with a few drops of stevia or a spoon of erythritol lets you control the final taste, adding just the right amount of sweetness without causing a dramatic rise in glucose. The result is a dessert that feels indulgent, rich, and indulgent — a perfect way to celebrate without straying from your health goals.

Or consider a creamy cheesecake made with an almond flour base. Traditionally, cheesecake relies on a buttery graham cracker crust and a rich mixture of cream cheese and sugar. Here, we substitute the base with ground almonds or a blend of almonds and coconut, adding texture and a nutty depth of flavor without the carbohydrate rush. The filling, made from cream cheese and a low-caloric sweetener, sets into a rich, smooth texture. A handful of strawberries or raspberries tossed on top brings color, tartness, and a touch of natural sweetness — a perfect contrast to the creamy base.

Flourless brownies, cookies, and lemon bars become viable and desirable alternatives when we employ ingredients like almonds, coconut flour, and dark chocolate. Instead of all-purpose flour, we use low-carbohydrate flours rich in fiber and healthy fats. Naturally sweetening these treats lets us cut back on excess carbohydrates without feeling deprived. The result is a rich, fudge-like brownie or a crispy-on-the-edges cookie that tastes indulgent and comforting — a perfect match for a warm cup of coffee or a chilled glass of unsweetened nut milk.

Peanut butter balls and "fat bombs" — small, rich treats made from a blend of nut butters, coconut oil, and dark chocolate — are another powerful tool in your ketogenic arsenal. They serve a dual purpose: satisfying a sweet or rich craving while delivering a convenient, energy-dense boost when you need it. Whether you roll them in chopped almonds or simply chill them into tiny cubes, these little delights keep you satiated and feeling indulgent without adding a large amount of carbohydrate.

Some of the most elegant and simple ketogenic desserts require no baking at all. Panna cotta — a silky, creamy Italian treat — is easily adapted to a ketogenic lifestyle by swapping the traditional sugar for a low-caloric sweetener and adding pure vanilla or a hint of berry. Coconut macaroons, made from shredded coconut, egg whites, and a touch of erythritol, come together quickly and bake into crispy-on-the-outside, tender-on-the-inside cookies — a perfect match for a rich cup of coffee or a warm mug of tea.

As you pursue this lifestyle, having a repertoire of ketogenic desserts lets you celebrate special occasions, treat yourself, and navigate holiday traditions without straying from your goals. Whether you're honoring a birthday, a promotion, or simply a dinner party with friends, you can serve something that feels festive and indulgent, while honoring your health. Importantly, these treats help diminish cravings over time, reducing the temptation to revert back to carbohydrate-rich sweets. Your taste buds gradually become more sensitive to natural flavors, letting you appreciate the rich notes of vanilla, chocolate, strawberries, and coconut — without needing a rush of refined sugar to find satisfaction.

This chapter comprises more than 20 recipes designed to suit all preferences and cooking skills. There are no-bake delights alongside rich, creamy classics; chilled sweets alongside warm, comforting treats. Whatever your mood or your cravings, you will find something here to match it — without derailing your progress. The key lies in choosing ingredients carefully, honoring both your health goals and your taste preferences.

Your ketogenic journey should be filled with indulgences — the kind that nourish you physically and satisfy you emotionally — a perfect blend of discipline and indulgence. The treats you'll discover here allow you to enjoy all the pleasures of food while honoring your goals, proving once and for all that you do not need to sacrifice taste or texture for health. Sweetness and health can coexist; rich flavor and discipline can walk hand in hand.

As you become more proficient in this lifestyle, you'll find yourself growing more creative in the kitchen, devising your own combinations of ingredients to suit your preferences. The ketogenic diet is not restrictive; it's a framework, a set of guidelines that help you nourish yourself while honoring your health goals. Within this framework, there is an extraordinary amount of freedom to innovate — to blend texture, flavor, and richness into a small plate or a festive dessert — and that's where these recipes become a powerful tool.

Picture a rich, velvety chocolate cheesecake made without a gram of added sugar — its base constructed from ground almonds and a touch of butter, yielding a crispy texture beneath a smooth, creamy filling. The filling itself, sweetened with a blend of erythritol and vanilla, delivers pure indulgence without adding to your carbohydrate load. The result is a sophisticated, satisfying dessert that you can serve to guests without a hint of guilt — or to yourself when you need a moment of indulgence in your day.

Flourless brownies, meanwhile, become a perfect blend of rich chocolate and fudge-like texture without a drop of conventional flour. The batter comes together quickly in a food processor, swapping all-purpose flour for a mixture of avocado, dark chocolate, and a small amount of nut meal. The result is a brownie that's dense and rich — perfect with a dollop of whipped cream or a handful of strawberries — a small piece delivering pure satisfaction without a dramatic rise in glucose.

The cookies you bake on a ketogenic diet can be surprisingly close to their traditional counterparts in texture and taste. The key lies in choosing the right base — blanched almonds or coconut flour — and adding a sweetener that performs well under heat. Erythritol is a popular choice here; it has a clean, sweet taste without the aftertaste that many associate with alternative sweeteners. Combine this with rich ingredients — dark chocolate chips, chopped pecans, or pure vanilla — and you have cookies that match their traditional ancestors in flavor, without the carbohydrate content that normally accompanies them.

Lemon bars — a classic treat — can be reinvented by swapping their shortbread base for a mixture of ground almonds and butter, and their tart lemon filling can be thickened without adding a large amount of carbohydrate. The result is a creamy, tangy, sweet treat — perfect for a summer afternoon — without a dramatic rise in glucose or a feeling of sluggishness afterwards.

Peanut butter balls, often called "fat bombs" in ketogenic circles, are a wonderful way to combine indulgence with practicality. They typically blend peanut or other nut butters with a small amount of sweetener and sometimes dark chocolate or coconut. Chilled, and then dipped in dark chocolate or chopped nuts, these small treats become rich, creamy, and satisfying — perfect for a midday energy boost or a small after-dinner indulgence.

Some of these sweets, like panna cotta, require no baking at all. Traditionally made by adding gelatin to a mixture of heavy cream and sweetener, panna cotta sets into a silky, smooth texture. Flavor it with vanilla, lemon, or a small amount of berry purée and you have a sophisticated, creamy dessert that's rich in texture and low in carbohydrates.

Coconut macaroons follow a similar path. Shredded coconut, a bit of sweetener, and whipped whites come together quickly and bake into crispy, sweet clusters — a perfect match for your afternoon coffee or a light dessert after dinner. The rich flavor of coconut naturally lends itself to a ketogenic lifestyle; it's rich in medium-chain triglycerides — a kind of fatty acid that converts quickly into energy — adding a functional health boost alongside pure indulgence.

Meanwhile, you can create a whole range of cheesecakes — from miniature cheesecake bites to large, dramatic cheesecakes — all without adding a traditional graham cracker base or refined sugar. Sweetening with erythritol or a small amount of stevia lets you control the final taste, while adding texture from ground almonds or pistachios. The result is a rich, creamy treat — perfect for a special dinner or a holiday meal — that highlights your ability to live a rich, full lifestyle while honoring your health goals.

Your ketogenic journey will be filled with these small triumphs — moments where you realize you're not deprived or stranded on a restrictive diet, but instead you're experiencing a rich world of food. The key is choosing ingredients that align with your health, swapping in healthy fats and low-carbohydrate components to produce something that feels indulgent, satisfying, and festive.

This approach transforms your relationship with food. Instead of feeling temptation or shame when you encounter a plate of cookies or a rich dessert, you become empowered to create your own versions — ones that align with your lifestyle and goals. There is a deep peace in this, a liberation from the oppressive diet culture that says health must come with suffering. Here, you learn that you can enjoy rich food without feeling guilty afterwards.

Your ability to appreciate these treats grows alongside your discipline. The more you practice choosing ingredients and designing recipes to suit your lifestyle, the more proficient you become at honoring both health and indulgence. Your taste buds become more sophisticated; you appreciate the pure, rich flavors of dark chocolate, strawberries, vanilla, and almonds — without needing a rush of refined sugar to activate your senses.

As you pursue this path, you will find yourself extending these techniques into all aspects of your cooking. Your main dishes become more colorful, your side dishes more rich and satisfying, and your snacks more purposeful and health-oriented. The discipline you apply here transforms not only your plate but your entire view of food. It ceases to be a battleground — a place where temptation wars against discipline — and instead becomes a rich canvas for creativity, indulgence, and nourishment.

CHAPTER 17 — INTERMITTENT FASTING EXPLAINED

In the rich and intricate journey toward health and transformation, there are combinations that emerge as profoundly powerful, adding dimensions of simplicity and depth to a lifestyle already designed to maximize well-being. Among these, the marriage of a ketogenic diet with intermittent fasting stands as a remarkable synergy — a way to further illuminate the path toward sustained energy, deep metabolic repair, and lasting change.

When we talk about intermittent fasting, we are not discussing a restrictive diet in the conventional sense, but a pattern of eating — a framework — that cycles between periods of nourishment and periods of abstinence. It's a practice that finds its roots in human physiology and ancestry; for millennia, humans lived without a constant supply of food, experiencing natural phases of scarcity and abundance. Our physiology is designed to handle these fluctuations gracefully, and when we align ourselves with this pattern, we activate mechanisms that can profoundly affect health and body composition.

This chapter aims to unveil how intermittent fasting, when combined with a ketogenic diet, can accelerate and deepen the metabolic shift you're already experiencing on your low-carbohydrate, high-fat regimen. At its core, this combination works by depleting your body's glucose stores more quickly and more thoroughly, thereby forcing a faster and more sustained production of ketones. Instead of primarily burning glucose for energy, your body transitions into a state where fatty acids become the main energy substrate. The result is a metabolic environment rich in ketones — a powerful alternative energy source — which can aid in unlocking numerous health benefits.

One of the most dramatic effects of this combination is its ability to break plateaus. If you find yourself stalling in your weight-loss journey, adding a fasting window can be the key to accessing those last few pounds or unlocking further progress. It assists in reducing calorie intake naturally, without the need for rigorous calorie counting or restrictive meal plans. Furthermore, by extending the period during which your insulin levels stay low, you enable your body to tap into its own fat stores more efficiently.

This process isn't just about physical transformation; it profoundly impacts the health of your cells. Fasting stimulates autophagy — a process of cellular renewal — where damaged components within your cells are identified, removed, and recycled. This assists in cleaning up faulty components and strengthening cellular structures, adding a layer of renewal to your health journey. Furthermore, this renewal has implications for metabolic disorders, neurodegenerative conditions, and the effects of aging.

Your body converts fatty acids into ketones more efficiently during a fast, which results in enhanced mental clarity and sustained energy. Instead of the fluctuations associated with a carbohydrate-centric diet — the rise and fall of blood sugar — you enjoy a stable and reliable flow of energy. Your mind feels sharper, your focus more sustained, and your physical activity less influenced by hunger signals.

There are numerous methods for implementing intermittent fasting alongside your ketogenic lifestyle. The most popular is the 16:8 method, which involves fasting for 16 hours and consuming all your calories within an 8-hour window. Some people opt for a 24-hour fast once or twice a week, while others may practice alternate-day fasting. The key is choosing a pattern that fits your lifestyle and preferences — there is no "one size fits all"— and honoring your body's signals.

Starting this journey safely and effectively is a crucial consideration. It's often wise to ease into the practice, extending your overnight fast by a few hours at first, then gradually extending it to 16 hours or more. Staying adequately hydrated, consuming enough sodium and other electrolytes, and honoring signals of true hunger are all important components of a successful transition.

Pairing a ketogenic diet with intermittent fasting is a powerful, flexible approach to health — a way to amplify the benefits you're already experiencing from reducing carbohydrates and shifting your body into a state of deep, sustained ketosis. The two strategies together create a synergy — a metabolic environment — that lets you efficiently tap into your body's own resources, repair and renewal mechanisms, and deep stores of energy.

This combination not only assists in weight-loss and metabolic health but also brings a range of secondary benefits — from improved mental clarity and reduced cravings to enhanced physical endurance and a greater sense of control over your eating habits. It reconnects you with a more ancestral pattern of nourishment and consumption — a pattern that, for much of human history, was the norm.

As you move forward, you may find that this approach transforms not just your physical health but your relationship with food, hunger, and nourishment itself. It invites you to appreciate the signals of your own body, to become more in tune with its needs and rhythms. It highlights a powerful principle — that sometimes, less can be more — and that a period of rest and renewal can be profoundly healing.

Your ketogenic journey, combined with intermittent fasting, has the potential to become a rich path to renewal — a way to reconnect with your body's natural ability to heal, repair, and flourish. Whether you pursue it daily or a few times a week, this powerful combination underscores the adaptability and resiliency that lie within you. It shows you that health is not a static state but a dynamic process — a delicate balance that, when supported by the right lifestyle choices, brings you back into harmony with your physiology and your greatest potential.

As you delve further into this combination of ketogenic lifestyle and intermittent fasting, you'll discover that it's not a rigid formula but a flexible tool — a way to respond to your body's signals and goals in real time. There may be days when you naturally gravitate toward a longer fast, feeling effortlessly satiated and strong without food, and there may be days when you shorten it to match your activity level or stress. The key is honoring these signals and understanding the physiology at play.

Your body is designed to be adaptable. It maintains health and balance by shifting its metabolic state in response to scarcity or abundance. Fasting lets you tap into this adaptability — it signals your body to maximize its resources, repair damage, and become more efficient in its energy utilization. That adaptability underpins many of the health benefits we associate with this lifestyle — reduced inflammation, improved insulin sensitivity, lower blood pressure, and a dramatic reduction in the risk of chronic disease — from diabetes and obesity to neurodegenerative disorders and certain forms of cancer.

Some people find, as their body adjusts to this combination of diet and fasting, their cravings diminish and their relationship with food evolves. The urgency to eat frequently drops away. Instead of feeling enslaved by hunger signals or blood sugar drops, you become more in control — choosing when and what to eat based on true nourishment needs instead of habit or temptation. This newfound freedom can be profoundly empowering, adding a psychological dimension to health that resonates far beyond the plate.

This synergy can be particularly helpful in addressing health issues related to metabolic dysfunction. Type 2 diabetes, obesity, fatty liver, and metabolic syndrome all reflect a body that has become less proficient at accessing its own energy stores and regulating its internal environment. Intermittent fasting, combined with a ketogenic diet, directly confronts these abnormalities by reducing the glucose load, improving insulin signaling, and lowering chronic inflammation. The result, for many, is dramatic and sustained health improvement — a reversal of conditions previously thought to be permanent or progressive.

Some practitioners find this approach helpful in slowing the effects of neurodegenerative disorders. The production of ketones during a fast, alongside reduced glucose availability, can provide an alternative energy to neurons, reducing their metabolic stress and improving their ability to repair and clear debris. There is growing research into this phenomenon, suggesting potential benefits for conditions such as Alzheimer's and Parkinson's disease.

Furthermore, this combination has a powerful role to play in reducing the risk of certain cancers and improving the body's ability to respond to stress and damage. The reduction in glucose, insulin, and growth signals during fasting can help slow the growth of rapidly dividing cells and induce protective mechanisms in healthy cells. Although this is a complex area of research and not a substitute for conventional treatments, it highlights a growing understanding of how lifestyle choices can influence disease progression and health at a deep, cellular level.

Your physical performance and recovery may also benefit from this approach. Athletes who practice intermittent fasting alongside a ketogenic diet often report greater metabolic flexibility — the ability to efficiently utilize both fatty acids and glucose — which can translate into enhanced endurance, faster recovery, and reduced muscle damage. Furthermore, the reduced inflammation associated with this lifestyle may help ease muscle soreness and joint discomfort, allowing for more consistent training and physical activity.

Sleep and stress, two key components of health, may also be positively influenced by this combination. Fasting has a powerful ability to stabilize circadian rhythms and promote deep, restful sleep — likely due to its effects on metabolic signals, growth factors, and stress hormones. Lowering chronic stress, reducing systemic inflammation, and improving metabolic health collectively create a physiology more conducive to relaxation and recovery. The result can be a dramatic improvement in energy, mood, and overall well-being.

Ultimately, this approach underscores a principle that we often forget in a world obsessed with constant consumption and excess: we are designed to flourish under conditions of scarcity and renewal. The human body is not a fragile machine; it is a resilient, adaptable ecosystem that performs optimally when challenged in healthy, purposeful ways — and then given the opportunity to repair and grow.

Pairing a ketogenic diet with intermittent fasting is a powerful expression of this principle. It signals your physiology to clear away what is weak or faulty and to fortify what is strong and useful. It lets you become more metabolically flexible, more resilient, more adaptable — not just physically, but mentally and emotionally — allowing you to navigate stress and change with greater ease.

As you move forward on this path, remember that there is no universal formula for health — only principles that you can apply to find what works best for you. Experiment with different fasting windows. Monitor how you feel, how you perform, and how your health evolves. Support your body's ability to heal by honoring its signals and honoring its remarkable adaptability.

Ultimately, this combination of ketogenic diet and intermittent fasting is not a punishment or a restrictive regimen; it's a powerful tool — a way to align your lifestyle with your physiology — unlocking health, energy, and renewal from within. It invites you to become an active participant in your own well-being, not a passive recipient of health care. It guides you back toward a more natural state — a state of metabolic health — where your body can do what it was designed to do: heal, repair, grow, and flourish.

CHAPTER 18 — TIPS FOR SUCCESSFUL FASTING

Walking the path of a ketogenic lifestyle is a rich, intimate journey — a transformation not just of your body but of your mind, your habits, and your future. Among the most powerful strategies you can employ on this path is intermittent fasting, a tool that, when mastered, can amplify all the benefits you're already experiencing from a low-carbohydrate diet. Fasting isn't about starving yourself; it's about letting your body do what it naturally wants to do when given a break from constant eating. It's a state of renewal, a period where your cells can clear away waste, repair damage, and become more efficient. But making this practice a comfortable, effective part of your lifestyle requires knowledge, preparation, and a few key strategies. That's exactly what this chapter aims to empower you with — a rich understanding of how to fast successfully and gracefully.

The first consideration when you embark on a fast is hydration. Your body depends on fluids not just for hydration but for numerous metabolic processes. During a fast, you're not consuming fluids from food, which typically comprises about 20% of your water intake. That means you need to be more conscious of drinking fluids directly. Water is your best friend here — pure, clear, and abundant — and adding a pinch of

Himalayan or sea salt to your water can help replenish sodium and other key electrolytes that may become temporarily imbalanced during your fast. Staying adequately hydrated will help ease symptoms of "keto flu"— weakness, headache, or muscle cramps — and will keep you feeling clear, strong, and comfortable.

Herbal tea is another wonderful tool during a fast. Naturally calorie-free, rich in antioxidants, and warm in a way that can be profoundly comforting, tea can ease hunger signals and make the hours pass more quickly. Black coffee is a popular aid during a fast, adding a bit of energy and a feeling of satiety without adding calories or breaking the fast's metabolic benefits. Nonetheless, it's a good idea to avoid adding cream or sweetener; black is best during a true fast.

Managing stress is another key consideration. Your body interprets stress signals as a form of danger, triggering the release of adrenaline and cortisol — two stress hormones — which can undermine your ability to remain in a fasted state. That's why relaxation techniques, deep breathing, and gentle movement — a walk in nature, some yoga, or simply sitting quietly — can be helpful in keeping stress under control and making your fast more comfortable. Staying busy is a powerful tactic against temptation; when you're engaged in something you love — reading a book, gardening, organizing your home — you're less likely to dwell on food and more likely to appreciate the clarity and lightness that come with an empty stomach.

Sleep plays a huge role in all of this. A restful night signals to your body that it's a time to repair and regenerate, not to scavenge for calories. Poor or interrupted sleep can undermine your ability to fast successfully by disturbing your hunger signals and making you more prone to temptation. Establishing a consistent bedtime, reducing caffeine in the afternoon, and avoiding screens in the evening can help you maximize rest and allow your body's natural rhythms to align with your fasting goals.

Some people find black coffee or plain tea to be helpful in blunting their appetite without adding calories. The bitter compounds in these drinks can act as a temporary appetite suppressant, making it easier to prolong the fast without discomfort. Nevertheless, it's important not to rely on caffeine to mask true signals from your body; it's meant to be a tool, not a crutch.

This chapter aims to empower you to navigate your fast successfully by understanding these signals — when you're experiencing true hunger and when you're simply battling temptation or habit — and by employing strategies to ease those moments. It guides you through choosing a fasting window that fits your lifestyle — whether it's a 16:8 fast, a 24-hour fast once a week, or something more advanced — and highlights the signals you should watch for, the small signs from your body that tell you when it's time to break your fast safely.

Breaking your fast is a delicate process. Ideally, you should ease back into eating with something rich in nutrients but gentle on your digestive system — a small serving of avocado, a handful of olives, or a bowl of bone broth. Eating a large meal immediately after a fast can overwhelm your digestive system and undermine some of the benefits you were meant to enjoy. So starting slow, honoring your body's signals of true hunger, and choosing foods that are rich in healthy fats, proteins, and micronutrients is key.

Your body adjusts quickly; what feels challenging at first soon becomes effortless. Fasting evolves from a temporary discipline into a powerful lifestyle tool — a way of honoring your body's ability to heal, cleanse, and regenerate. It lets you break free from the tyranny of constant snacking and learn to appreciate food in a new, more intimate context.

This chapter aims to empower you with knowledge, confidence, and a deep understanding of the physiology of fasting. It guides you toward making choices that align with your health goals and help you realize the full potential of a ketogenic lifestyle combined with intermittent fasting. The result is a powerful synergy — a state where you become a proficient, flexible, resilient, and profoundly healthy human being.

As you progress further into this lifestyle, you'll discover something remarkable: the discipline of fasting starts to permeate all aspects of your health and well-being. It's not just about reducing calories or losing a few pounds; it's about honoring your body's ability to regulate itself, heal, and become more efficient. Your cells, when given a break from constant nourishment, activate a process called autophagy — a kind of deep cleaning, a renewal from within. During autophagy, damaged components are removed and recycled, making room for healthy, strong components to flourish. It's this process that underpins many of the health benefits associated with intermittent fasting — from reduced inflammation and improved metabolic health to enhanced resistance to stress and disease.

This renewal isn't instantaneous; it evolves gracefully, over hours and days without food. That's why extending your fast from a simple 16 hours to a 24-hour fast once or twice a week can profoundly deepen these benefits. Your body enters a state of deep repair and renewal, consuming components it no longer needs and strengthening its ability to resist future stressors. Importantly, this process signals your body to release growth factors and activate genes associated with longevity and resiliency. The result is not just a thinner you, but a more robust, youthful, and adaptable you.

Managing temptation during these longer fasts can be challenging at first, but it's a challenge you can conquer. Staying busy and engaged is key; when your mind is occupied, you're less prone to thinking about food. Activities that absorb you — reading, gardening, creative hobbies — become powerful allies in maintaining your fast without discomfort. Support from friends or family who appreciate your health journey can be a huge help, adding a layer of encouragement and understanding when temptation strikes.

Your hydration strategies become even more important during longer fasts. Continuing to drink fluids and adding a small amount of Himalayan or sea salt to your water can help maintain electrolyte balance and avoid weakness or headaches. Black coffee or plain tea remain helpful in keeping your energy and focus, provided you consume them in reasonable amounts. Some people find that adding a drop of apple cider vinegar to water can help ease cravings and stabilize blood sugar, adding to their ability to fast gracefully.

Sleep, rest, and relaxation become powerful components of your regimen during a longer fast. Your body is busy internally, conducting repairs and renewal. Providing it with rest — through naps, relaxation techniques, and a good night's sleep — lets these processes unfold unhindered. It's a time to appreciate your body's ability to heal and reset itself, and honoring that ability by resting deeply is a key part of a successful fast.

When it comes time to break your fast, choosing the right foods can be the difference between feeling great and feeling bloated or sick. Naturally, you should avoid heavy, rich, or hard-to-digest foods immediately after a fast. Instead, opt for something light and rich in nutrients — a small serving of avocado, a warm bowl of bone broth, a handful of olives — something gentle and easy to assimilate. After 30-60 minutes, you can progress to a more substantial meal — a piece of grilled fatty fish or a salad tossed in olive oil — honoring your ketogenic lifestyle while honoring your body's signals.

Your ability to fast successfully will grow with practice. At first, you may find it challenging to miss a meal or two. But soon you will appreciate the lightness and clarity that come from not always having to eat, from trusting your body to provide its own energy and renewal. The discipline you develop through intermittent fasting will permeate other aspects of your life, strengthening your resolve, adding clarity to your goals, and deepening your understanding of what true nourishment means.

This powerful combination — a ketogenic diet rich in healthy fats and low in carbohydrates, teamed with intermittent fasting — lets you become a master of your own physiology. It lets you break free from cravings, from energy swings, and from the oppressive feeling of always needing to eat. It converts you from a person enslaved by food signals into a person who controls their own destiny — a person who lets their body determine when it wants nourishment and when it prefers renewal.

Your health, your energy, your clarity — all are profoundly influenced by this marriage of diet and lifestyle. The discipline you learn here will empower you in countless other endeavors, adding a deep confidence that you can conquer obstacles, resist temptation, and pursue goals that previously seemed unreachable. The knowledge you acquire — about your body, about the signals it emits, about the power you have over your own health — is a lifelong asset, something you will carry forward for years to come.

As you move forward on this path, remember to be kind to yourself. There will be days when you break a fast early or find it hard to avoid temptation. That's normal; it's human. The key is patience, persistence, and a deep understanding that you are not defined by a single meal or a single decision. Your progress is made by the sum of your choices, day after day. Each fast, each meal, each moment of discipline brings you closer to the health and freedom you seek.

CHAPTER 19 — COMBINING KETO AND FASTING SAFELY

There's a powerful synergy waiting for you at the intersection of two remarkable lifestyle strategies — the ketogenic diet and intermittent fasting. Individually, each has a rich legacy of health benefits backed by growing scientific understanding. Together, when done safely and with proper knowledge, their effects can be profoundly transformational. Here we will journey deep into how these two approaches amplify each other's benefits, accelerate your progress, and help you become a more energetic, resilient, and healthy person.

Picture your body as a finely tuned hybrid vehicle — a sophisticated machine designed to produce energy efficiently under a range of conditions. Naturally, we predominantly rely on glucose for energy; it's the fastest, most readily available form of fuel when we eat frequently and consume a diet rich in carbohydrates. But when we cut back on carbohydrates and allow ourselves periods without food — through a combination of ketogenic diet and intermittent fasting — we activate an alternative, powerful metabolic state called ketosis.

Ketosis occurs when your body starts breaking down its own fatty acids into ketone bodies, an efficient and sustainable form of energy. It's a process hardwired into human physiology, a backup plan meant for periods of scarcity or reduced food intake. The result isn't weakness and lethargy, but a remarkable renewal of energy, mental clarity, and physical stability — a state in which your body becomes proficient at tapping its own resources.

When you combine a ketogenic diet — which naturally depletes your glycogen stores — with periods of intermittent fasting — which further prolongs the time you abstain from consuming calories — you allow your body to enter and deepen this state more quickly and profoundly. The result is enhanced fat-burning, reduced cravings, and greater mental clarity — a powerful combination for those trying to lose excess weight, reverse metabolic dysfunction, or simply perform at their best.

Some people find their weight-loss plateaus when following a ketogenic diet on its own. That's because, over time, the body adapts to a new baseline and starts conserving energy. But when you introduce intermittent fasting into your regimen — extending the periods between your last meal and your first meal the following day — you create a further metabolic stress. It signals your body to release additional fatty acids from storage and produce more ketones to meet its energy needs.

This synergy can be profoundly helpful for breaking through plateaus and unlocking a new phase of progress. Furthermore, many people report reduced cravings and a dramatic improvement in their relationship with food when employing both strategies together. Without constant fluctuations in blood sugar and insulin, your body settles into a more stable metabolic rhythm. It no longer signals you to eat frequently, and you find yourself feeling satiated and clearheaded for hours on end.

Of course, the combination of ketogenic diet and intermittent fasting isn't something you should rush into without consideration. Your health conditions, medication regimen, lifestyle, and stress levels all affect your readiness to implement these strategies safely. If you are new to a low-carbohydrate diet, it's often a good idea to first become comfortable with ketogenic eating — dialing back your carbohydrate intake and allowing your body to become proficient at utilizing ketones — before adding intermittent fasting into your routine.

This gradual approach lets your body adjust without adding additional stress. Once you're proficient at burning fat for energy, extending your overnight fast or adding a 16:8 regimen — 16 hours of fasting followed by an 8-hour eating window — feels more natural and less challenging. Your body will already be in a state of low insulin and reduced glucose dependence, making the transition smoother.

Your health conditions should be taken into consideration. If you have diabetes, are taking medication for high blood pressure, or have a history of disordered eating, it's especially important to pursue this combination under the supervision of a health professional. Certain medication dosages may need to be lowered to avoid complications, and some health conditions may warrant a more gradual approach. Nonetheless, many people with metabolic disorders find this combination profoundly helpful in improving their health markers — from reducing their blood glucose and Hemoglobin A1c to improving their lipid profiles and reducing medication dependence — when done safely and under supervision.

Your lifestyle matters, too. If you are under a great deal of stress, frequently travel across time zones, or find it hard to control meal timing due to your responsibilities, it may be wiser to ease into this regimen. Begin by focusing on your diet first; cut back on carbohydrates, increase healthy fats, and allow your body to become a proficient fat burner. Once you find a comfortable baseline, you can start extending your overnight fast and seeing how your body responds. The key is patience — honoring your body's signals and making adjustments when necessary.

Ultimately, this approach is a powerful path toward health transformation when done safely and strategically. It lets you become a more efficient, flexible, and adaptable human, less prone to the fluctuations in energy, cravings, and mood that come from a carbohydrate-dominant diet. It strengthens your ability to rely on your own resources and deep metabolic reserves, making you less dependent on constant food intake.

As you progress, you will discover a newfound freedom. Your relationship with food will become more intuitive and less restrictive. Instead of battling hunger, you will learn to appreciate periods of emptiness and renewal. Your body will respond by letting go of excess weight, improving health markers, and experiencing greater mental clarity.

This isn't a short cut or a diet you follow for a few weeks; it's a powerful lifestyle, a way of honoring your physiology and unlocking its potential. There is a deep peace in understanding that your body is designed to do this — to produce energy efficiently, to heal, to cleanse, and to repair — when given the opportunity.

As you move forward with this combination, you'll find it touching nearly all aspects of health — from your physical appearance and metabolic health to your mental clarity and overall sense of well-being. The marriage of ketogenic diet and intermittent fasting is not a restrictive discipline; it's a powerful framework for honoring your body's physiology and unlocking its ability to heal, perform, and flourish.

Your body is designed to respond to scarcity gracefully. Traditionally, humans lived in an environment where food was not available at all hours of the day. There were periods of plenty — after a successful hunt or harvest — and periods of scarcity — when food was hard to come by. Our physiology evolves to handle these fluctuations efficiently. During scarcity, the body switches from a predominantly glucose-fueled state to a fatty acid- and ketone-fueled state. It starts breaking down its own resources — first from storage in the liver and muscles, then from its abundant reserve in body fat — to generate energy.

This ability to produce energy internally meant our ancestors were not weak or vulnerable during periods without food; in many cases, they were at their most mentally sharp and physically resilient. They were able to travel long distances in search of food, pursue game, and find water. Furthermore, this metabolic state triggered a range of repair mechanisms — from autophagy, which clears damaged components from cells, to reduced oxidative stress and inflammation — all contributing to renewal and maintenance.

When we combine ketogenic diet and intermittent fasting in a modern context, we're accessing these powerful mechanisms in a gentle, controllable way. The low carbohydrate intake signals to your body that glucose is scarce; the subsequent period of fasting then deepens this state, allowing a complete metabolic shift toward using fatty acids and ketones.

This synergy brings a cascade of health benefits. Your blood sugar drops and stabilises, reducing the stress on your pancreas and improving your insulin sensitivity. Your body starts breaking down its own stores of excess fat, not from a place of alarm or weakness, but from a state of metabolic confidence — a ability to produce energy from within. Furthermore, this process reduces chronic low-grade inflammation — a key driver of many lifestyle diseases — and clears away worn-out components through autophagy, making your cells more youthful and resilient.

Some people find this combination particularly helpful for addressing metabolic disorders such as obesity, Type 2 diabetes, and metabolic syndrome. Furthermore, many report a dramatic reduction in cravings and a newfound ability to appreciate food without feeling enslaved by it. It's not unusual for people to find their "food noise"— the constant thinking about what to eat and when — diminish profoundly once their physiology settles into this state.

This quietening of cravings is a direct result of stabilizing your blood sugar and honoring your body's ability to produce energy from its own stores. Without dramatic drops and surges in glucose, the signals that normally drive hunger become less pronounced. Furthermore, ketones — particularly beta-hydroxybutyrate — have a direct, satiating effect on the brain, dampening the release of the hunger hormone ghrelin and reducing the appeal of calorie-dense, processed foods.

This makes it much easier to practice fasting without feeling deprived and to make food choices that align with health goals instead of impulsive desires. Importantly, this process develops a sense of control and confidence in oneself — a deep understanding that you are not powerless against cravings or a slow metabolism; you have within you all the resources you need to become healthy, energetic, and strong.

CHAPTER 20 — HYDRATION, SUPPLEMENTS, AND SUPPORT

Embarking on a ketogenic journey is not simply about the foods you eat; it's a holistic transformation that touches every facet of your lifestyle. Among the often-underestimated pillars of keto success are hydration, the right supplementation, and having a supportive community standing with you through every twist and turn. Without these vital elements, even the most meticulously planned keto diet can falter, leaving you feeling fatigued, frustrated, or simply out of sync with your body's needs. This chapter is dedicated to unraveling the critical role these factors play and showing you how to weave them seamlessly into your daily routine for lasting transformation.

Water is life, and on a ketogenic diet, it becomes your closest ally. When you cut carbohydrates, your body sheds water weight rapidly in the initial days. Glycogen, the stored form of carbohydrate in muscles and liver, holds water molecules tightly; as glycogen depletes, water flushes out, often leading to a noticeable drop on the scale. But this rapid water loss can also create a risk: dehydration. You might feel lightheaded, tired, or notice muscle cramps if you don't drink enough. The body's need for water increases, not only because of this initial flush but also because fat metabolism itself produces more metabolic waste that requires flushing out through your kidneys. Keeping a steady, generous intake of water helps you stay energized, clear-headed, and supports your kidneys in their crucial detoxification role.

But hydration isn't just about water. On keto, your body's balance of electrolytes shifts dramatically. Electrolytes — primarily sodium, potassium, and magnesium — are essential minerals that conduct electrical signals in your body, regulating muscle contractions, nerve function, and fluid balance. When carbohydrate intake drops, insulin levels decline, and your kidneys excrete more sodium. This sodium loss triggers a chain reaction causing your body to shed potassium and magnesium as well. The result? You might experience what's commonly called the "keto flu," characterized by headaches, fatigue, nausea, and muscle cramps. These symptoms are often a cry for electrolyte replenishment.

To avoid these pitfalls, it's critical to proactively maintain your electrolyte balance. This means not just drinking water but also consciously including sodium in your diet through natural sources like bone broth, salted nuts, olives, and even adding a pinch of Himalayan or sea salt to your meals or water. Potassium is abundant in leafy greens, avocados, and nuts, while magnesium can be found in pumpkin seeds, spinach, and dark chocolate. In some cases, a quality magnesium supplement may be warranted to support restful sleep and reduce muscle cramps. These minerals are not optional extras; they are the foundation of your physical comfort and metabolic efficiency during keto adaptation.

Beyond hydration and electrolytes, supplementation can bridge nutritional gaps that naturally occur when you shift your eating habits. While a well-formulated ketogenic diet focuses on nutrient-dense, whole foods, certain vitamins and fatty acids are harder to obtain in optimal amounts. For example, omega-3 fatty acids, especially EPA and DHA, are vital for cardiovascular health, brain function, and reducing inflammation. Wild-caught fatty fish like salmon and mackerel are excellent sources, but if you don't consume them regularly, an omega-3 supplement derived from fish oil or algae can be invaluable.

Fiber is another area where supplementation might help. Low-carb vegetables provide some fiber, but if your digestion becomes sluggish, a fiber supplement can support gut health, regularity, and a balanced microbiome. Look for soluble fibers like psyllium husk or acacia fiber that won't interfere with ketosis. Similarly, some people benefit from a daily multivitamin to cover the bases — especially vitamins D and B-complex — but it's always best to get nutrients from whole foods whenever possible.

While hydration and supplements fortify your body, the social and emotional dimension of support fortifies your mindset. Embarking on a keto lifestyle can feel isolating, especially if your friends and family don't share your enthusiasm or knowledge. Yet, connection and encouragement are key to long-term success. Being part of a community where people understand your goals, share your struggles, and celebrate your victories can provide motivation when self-doubt creeps in or when the road gets bumpy.

Support can come from many places — in-person groups, online forums, social media communities, or even a trusted accountability partner. These networks offer a space to ask questions, exchange recipe ideas, discuss challenges like "keto flu" or intermittent fasting, and share personal milestones. They remind you that keto isn't a solitary endeavor but a shared journey with many who have walked the path before you. Moreover, hearing stories of others' transformations can spark your own resolve and creativity, helping you navigate plateaus or make your meals more exciting.

Your progress is greatly enhanced when you combine a solid hydration routine, thoughtful supplementation, and a vibrant support system. Together, they help you avoid common pitfalls, reduce discomfort, and build resilience — physically and mentally. Listening to your body's signals remains paramount. Some days you'll need more water, others might call for extra magnesium, and sometimes emotional encouragement is exactly what you need to keep pushing forward. By tuning into these needs, you align your lifestyle with your goals, creating a sustainable, rewarding ketogenic experience.

Integrating hydration, supplementation, and support isn't about perfection; it's about consistency and responsiveness. Your body and mind thrive when nurtured with intention, and the ketogenic lifestyle offers a profound opportunity for healing and transformation. Embrace these tools as part of your daily routine, and you'll find that your energy soars, your cravings diminish, and your commitment deepens. This is the foundation on which lasting health and vitality are built.

As you move forward, keep a water bottle close at hand, choose whole foods rich in electrolytes, consider supplements thoughtfully, and surround yourself with like-minded individuals who inspire and uplift you. The keto path is a marathon, not a sprint, and these essentials ensure you are well-equipped for every step. Your journey is not just about what you eat; it's about how you care for your entire being, mind and body, supported by knowledge and community. This holistic approach transforms not only your body composition but your relationship with food, health, and self-care itself. Welcome to the empowered, hydrated, and connected world of ketogenic living.

Continuing on this path, it's important to recognize that hydration needs can fluctuate daily depending on your activity level, climate, and even the phase of your ketogenic journey. In the beginning, as your body adapts to burning fat for fuel, you may find thirst increases, and your electrolyte demands shift rapidly. Listening closely to your body's subtle cues—dry mouth, dark urine, headaches, or muscle cramps—can guide you in adjusting your water intake and electrolyte supplementation accordingly. Over time, as your metabolism stabilizes, these needs often become more predictable, allowing you to fine-tune your personal hydration strategy.

Beyond just drinking water, consider incorporating mineral-rich beverages such as herbal teas or mineral water. Herbal teas, especially those with anti-inflammatory properties like ginger or peppermint, can soothe digestion and provide hydration without interrupting ketosis. Mineral water, naturally loaded with magnesium and calcium, can serve as a dual hydration and supplementation source. However, be mindful of beverages containing artificial sweeteners or hidden carbs, which can hinder your progress.

When it comes to supplementation, quality matters immensely. Not all supplements are created equal; choosing products that are third-party tested and free from fillers or unnecessary additives is crucial. For example, omega-3 supplements sourced from sustainably harvested fish or algae ensure purity and potency. Magnesium supplements come in various forms—magnesium citrate, glycinate, or oxide—each with different absorption rates and effects on digestion. Experimentation may be necessary to find what suits your body best, but consulting a healthcare professional can provide personalized guidance.

In addition to individual supplements, some ketogenic practitioners find benefit in using exogenous ketones during the early phases or plateaus of their diet. These supplements supply ketone bodies directly, potentially easing the transition into ketosis and supporting mental focus. However, they are not a substitute for proper diet and hydration but rather an adjunct for some individuals.

A particularly powerful aspect of support comes from shared knowledge and collective experience. When you engage with communities—whether through local meetups, online groups, or social media platforms—you tap into a reservoir of practical tips, troubleshooting advice, and emotional encouragement. Hearing how others overcame carb cravings, managed social events, or dealt with keto flu can arm you with strategies that prevent common setbacks. Sharing your own successes and challenges not only reinforces your commitment but helps others on similar paths.

Accountability plays a subtle but potent role here. When you know others are tracking their progress alongside you, checking in regularly, or celebrating milestones, you naturally become more consistent and motivated. This mutual encouragement fosters a sense of belonging and shared purpose, which is invaluable in sustaining long-term lifestyle changes. Beyond motivation, these connections often become sources of genuine friendship and support that extend far beyond the ketogenic diet itself.

It is also essential to maintain open communication with your healthcare provider, especially if you have pre-existing conditions or are taking medications. Some supplements or dietary shifts may interact with medications or require monitoring of blood markers. Your health team can help tailor your hydration, supplementation, and dietary approach to best support your individual physiology and goals.

As you cultivate this triad of hydration, supplementation, and support, remember that your body is remarkably adaptive. It responds not only to what you eat but how you nurture it emotionally and physically. By honoring its signals, being proactive in self-care, and surrounding yourself with a community that understands your journey, you create an environment where transformation becomes not just possible but inevitable.

Ultimately, ketogenic living is a celebration of empowerment — the empowerment to choose foods that fuel you, to listen deeply to your body's needs, and to embrace a supportive network that lifts you higher. Hydration, supplements, and social support are not just add-ons; they are foundational pillars that uphold your health, happiness, and sustainable success.

Step into this chapter as a guide to mastering these essentials, and carry this wisdom forward with confidence and grace. The path ahead is illuminated not only by what you put on your plate but by how you nurture your entire being and the connections you build along the way. Your ketogenic lifestyle is richer, fuller, and more rewarding because of it.

CHAPTER 21 — STAYING KETO ON THE GO

Embarking on the ketogenic journey is transformative, but the true test of dedication often comes when you're away from the comfort of your own kitchen—traveling through unfamiliar cities, sitting down at restaurant tables, or navigating the unpredictable environment of airports and road trips. This chapter delves deeply into how to maintain your ketogenic lifestyle on the go, turning potential challenges into opportunities for triumph rather than moments of defeat. The key is preparation, awareness, and adaptability, which empower you to make smart choices that keep you on track without feeling deprived or overwhelmed.

When you step out into the world, one of the first strategies to embrace is thoughtful planning. Before you head to a restaurant, attend a conference, or set off on a journey, take the time to research menus online. Nowadays, most restaurants offer their menus on their websites, and many even label low-carb or keto-friendly dishes. This simple step can eliminate a lot of stress before you arrive. Knowing where you can find grilled steak, fresh fish, or succulent chicken dishes allows you to focus on the experience rather than scrambling to find something suitable once you're there.

Protein-rich dishes naturally dominate many menus, which is a major advantage for keto adherents. Ordering grilled or roasted meats and seafood gives you a solid foundation of protein and fat, the building blocks of your ketogenic diet. When you receive your plate, make a conscious decision to remove starchy sides such as potatoes, rice, or bread, which are common traps for carbohydrates. Instead, ask if you can substitute these with non-starchy vegetables, like sautéed spinach, asparagus, or a side salad dressed in olive oil or butter. These swaps maintain your carb count low while keeping the meal filling and nutrient-dense.

Hidden carbohydrates lurk in places you might not expect, especially in sauces, dressings, and gravies. Many restaurants add sugar, flour, or cornstarch to enhance flavor and texture, turning a seemingly safe meal into a carb-heavy one. Become a detective when ordering—ask for sauces and dressings on the side, or better yet, request simple preparations like olive oil and vinegar or a lemon wedge. Don't hesitate to inquire about ingredients or preparation methods; chefs and servers are increasingly aware of dietary preferences and can often accommodate your needs with little fuss.

Carrying convenient snacks is another cornerstone of success when you're away from home. Airports, gas stations, and convenience stores can be carbohydrate minefields, filled with chips, candy, and processed foods designed for quick energy but laden with sugars and starches. Packing your own keto-friendly snacks ensures that hunger never forces you into poor choices. Portable options like beef jerky, almonds, macadamia nuts, string cheese, or even small containers of guacamole provide satisfying nutrition that fuels your body while keeping you firmly in ketosis. These snacks are easy to store, non-perishable for short trips, and can be your safety net during long flights or unexpected delays.

For longer journeys, meal prepping becomes your secret weapon. Preparing meals in advance that travel well—such as keto-friendly egg muffins, salads with olive oil dressing, or cold cuts paired with cheese—can save time and reduce stress. Portion these into containers that fit your travel bag, and you'll be ready to eat well no matter where your adventure takes you. Meal prep not only guarantees you stay within your macro limits but also helps you avoid the temptation to grab the fastest, most convenient, and often carb-laden option.

Sometimes, despite the best preparation, the options can feel limited. This chapter equips you with a series of quick fixes and hacks for such moments. For example, if you find yourself at a fast-food restaurant, many chains now offer bunless burgers or grilled chicken salads. Removing bread or tortilla shells immediately cuts down carbs, and choosing full-fat dressings or adding avocado can boost fat intake. When limited to convenience stores, look for nuts, cheese sticks, hard-boiled eggs, or even canned sardines or tuna, all keto staples that require no preparation. Hydrating well with water or sparkling water keeps you feeling full and curbs hunger pangs between meals.

Navigating social gatherings, business dinners, or family events adds another layer of complexity, but it's far from impossible. Communicate your dietary preferences confidently but politely, and often people will be more accommodating than you expect. Offer to bring a keto-friendly dish to share—this ensures there's something you can eat while introducing others to delicious low-carb alternatives. Remember that your ability to stay ketogenic under all circumstances doesn't just reflect discipline; it reflects your commitment to your health, your goals, and your well-being.

The flexibility and adaptability you develop through these experiences build resilience. Being able to stick to your ketogenic lifestyle despite being in new or challenging environments strengthens your resolve and confidence. It turns the diet from a restrictive chore into a sustainable, enjoyable lifestyle choice that fits naturally with your day-to-day life. It means that wherever you are—whether on a bustling city street, a quiet country road, or the terminal of an international airport—you can thrive.

Ultimately, mastering the art of staying keto on the go is about embracing empowerment through preparation and knowledge. It's about making informed choices, setting realistic expectations, and trusting yourself to navigate the inevitable hurdles. This chapter guides you not only with practical tips and meal ideas but also with the mindset needed to succeed. When you blend smart planning with flexibility, you make your ketogenic lifestyle not just a diet, but a way of life that travels with you, wherever you may go.

As you deepen your journey, you'll find that staying keto on the go becomes second nature. You learn to read menus like a pro, identifying carb traps and hidden sugars effortlessly. Your palate adapts, finding satisfaction in the rich flavors of fats and proteins rather than relying on carbs for comfort. The confidence gained from successfully navigating restaurants, social occasions, and travel environments translates into a powerful sense of autonomy and control over your health.

Being proactive also means anticipating challenges before they arise. For example, long travel days can disrupt your meal timing and hydration. Carrying a refillable water bottle and electrolyte supplements can keep you balanced and energized throughout the day. Bringing a small cooler or insulated bag for perishable keto snacks can make a huge difference, especially when airport security or customs regulations might prevent you from bringing certain foods inside.

When dining out, don't shy away from customizing your order. Requesting extra butter, cheese, or avocado not only enhances the flavor but also increases your fat intake, which is crucial for staying in ketosis. Opt for cooking methods like grilling, roasting, or sautéing in healthy fats rather than fried or breaded preparations. Over time, you develop a natural instinct for modifying dishes to suit your needs without making the experience feel like a compromise.

Socially, being keto on the go also means managing expectations and sometimes educating those around you. Sharing your reasons for choosing this lifestyle, such as better energy, mental clarity, or health improvements, can inspire curiosity and support. When friends or colleagues understand your commitment, they are more likely to offer accommodations or join you in low-carb choices.

On the road, being keto doesn't mean missing out on new culinary experiences. Many cultures offer naturally low-carb options—such as grilled meats and fresh vegetables in Mediterranean cuisine, sushi sashimi without rice in Japanese fare, or rich curries in Indian cooking served with cauliflower rice. Exploring these dishes expands your culinary repertoire and keeps your meals exciting.

Another critical aspect of staying keto while traveling is managing unexpected cravings or indulgences. The occasional treat may happen, and that's okay. What matters is how you respond afterward. Returning to your regular eating pattern quickly prevents setbacks and reinforces your long-term habits. This flexible approach makes your ketogenic lifestyle more sustainable and less stressful.

Mindset plays a crucial role as well. Viewing your ketogenic lifestyle as a positive, empowering choice rather than a restrictive diet fosters resilience and joy. Embrace the journey, celebrate small victories, and remind yourself why you chose this path. Staying keto on the go isn't just about the food; it's about the freedom and vitality that come with making choices that honor your body's needs.

By mastering these strategies, you unlock a new level of freedom—one where your health goals and your lifestyle coexist harmoniously, no matter where life takes you. Your ketogenic lifestyle becomes not a limitation but a launchpad for better energy, sharper focus, and vibrant wellbeing, carried confidently in your suitcase, backpack, or purse.

This chapter equips you not just with practical tools but with the mindset and resilience to thrive. Wherever you travel, whatever meal you face, you have the knowledge and confidence to make choices that nourish your body and soul. The road ahead is yours to navigate—keto on the go is no longer a challenge, but a celebration of your commitment to living well, on your terms.

CHAPTER 22 — DINING OUT TIPS AND TRICKS

Dining out while following a ketogenic lifestyle can seem like a daunting task at first, but with the right mindset and strategies, it becomes an empowering opportunity rather than a stressful challenge. Eating away from home often brings concerns about hidden carbohydrates, sauces laden with sugars, and the ever-present temptation of bread baskets and carb-heavy sides. However, understanding how to navigate menus, communicate clearly with restaurant staff, and make smart, keto-friendly choices can transform dining out into an enjoyable experience that complements your ketogenic journey rather than sabotages it.

At the heart of successful keto dining out is knowledge and assertiveness. Asking the right questions to your server or chef can unlock a world of options that might otherwise remain hidden beneath menus crafted for more conventional eating habits. When you engage with your server, don't hesitate to inquire about how dishes are prepared — specifically requesting details about ingredients and cooking methods. Many kitchens use hidden sugars, breading, or starches in seemingly innocent dishes. By proactively asking if sauces contain flour or sugar, whether meats are breaded or marinated in sugary mixtures, and if the vegetables are cooked with butter or oil rather than starchy sauces, you gain a clearer picture of what is safe to order.

Customizing your order is one of the most effective tactics in dining out keto. Removing buns from burgers, swapping fries for a fresh side salad, or asking for sauces on the side can drastically reduce your carbohydrate intake while allowing you to enjoy your meal fully. You have the right to modify dishes to meet your nutritional goals, and most restaurants are happy to accommodate special requests when approached politely and clearly. This proactive approach prevents accidental carb overload, helps maintain your ketosis, and empowers you to take charge of your dietary choices in any environment.

Certain cuisines naturally lend themselves better to ketogenic eating. Mexican food, for example, offers many keto-friendly options when you skip the tortillas and rice. Grilled meats, fajitas without the shells, and fresh guacamole with sour cream make for satisfying, high-fat, low-carb meals. Mediterranean cuisine is another excellent choice, often featuring olive oils, fatty fish, cheeses, and fresh vegetables that fit seamlessly into keto macros. Steakhouses are particularly friendly for keto diners, as their menus typically revolve around high-quality cuts of meat and non-starchy sides such as steamed greens, asparagus, or sautéed mushrooms.

Despite these options, some restaurants will be more restrictive than others. Fast-food chains or places heavily focused on carb-rich dishes might not offer many keto-compliant choices. In such cases, it's wise to plan ahead by reviewing menus online or calling ahead to check what keto-friendly options exist. Preparation eliminates last-minute stress and ensures you won't be caught off guard by limited selections. Alternatively, you can adapt by focusing on the protein component and pairing it with simple, keto-friendly sides you can carry with you, such as nuts or cheese sticks.

Balancing your meal with non-starchy vegetables is a crucial component of dining out on keto. Sides like sautéed spinach, kale, broccoli, or cauliflower rice are nutritious and fit well within ketogenic macros, providing fiber and micronutrients without tipping your carbohydrate intake over the edge. When ordering, make these veggies your go-to choices instead of high-carb alternatives like potatoes, rice, or bread. This small swap helps you feel full, satisfied, and confident that you are staying on track with your goals.

One of the most important attitudes you can adopt is being unapologetically assertive about your dietary needs. It's your health and well-being on the line, so don't be shy about making requests or clarifying doubts. Many restaurant staff appreciate customers who communicate clearly about allergies or dietary restrictions because it helps them deliver a better experience. By standing firm on your keto requirements, you reinforce your commitment to yourself and your lifestyle. This self-advocacy often opens doors to customized meal preparations and builds your confidence in handling social dining situations.

Understanding that you have control over your choices is a powerful mindset shift. Restaurants exist to serve their customers, and your requests for substitutions or ingredient clarifications are part of that dynamic. You can guide the kitchen to create dishes that nourish your body, satisfy your palate, and keep your metabolism in fat-burning mode. This empowerment transforms dining out from a potential threat to ketosis into a reaffirmation of your keto commitment.

Dining out on a ketogenic diet doesn't have to be a compromise or an occasional indulgence fraught with guilt. With thoughtful preparation, clear communication, and an understanding of your food choices, your meals away from home can be just as delicious, fulfilling, and aligned with your goals as those prepared in your own kitchen. This chapter encourages you to embrace dining out as part of your ketogenic lifestyle, knowing that every meal can be a celebration of health, flavor, and personal empowerment.

Navigating the world of restaurants with a ketogenic lens also means learning to read between the lines of menus. Many dishes will be described in ways that obscure their carbohydrate content. Words like "glazed," "breaded," "crispy," or "marinated" can hint at hidden sugars or flours. Don't hesitate to ask for details or suggest alternatives. For example, if a salad comes with candied nuts or dried fruits, ask if those can be omitted, and request extra olive oil or avocado to maintain your fat intake.

When it comes to beverages, water should always be your first choice. Avoid sugary sodas, fruit juices, and sweetened teas. If you prefer something flavorful, sparkling water with a wedge of lemon or lime provides refreshment without carbs. Coffee and tea are usually safe, but beware of added sugar or flavored creamers. Many coffee shops now offer unsweetened nut milks or heavy cream as options, allowing you to enjoy your caffeine fix without breaking your fast or ketosis.

Alcohol can be tricky, as many drinks contain sugars and carbohydrates that can kick you out of ketosis. However, dry wines, spirits like vodka or whiskey (served neat or with soda water), and light beer in moderation can fit into your ketogenic lifestyle. Always check with your server about mixers and ingredients to avoid hidden sugars.

Another useful tip is to embrace the idea of "protein first." Prioritize ordering quality protein sources such as grilled chicken, steak, or fish, and then build the meal around those choices. By focusing on protein and fat, you satisfy hunger and keep your metabolic engine running efficiently. Adding fats like butter, olive oil, or avocado can help you reach your macro goals while keeping carbs low.

For special occasions or celebrations where dining out is inevitable and choices may be limited, consider eating a keto-friendly snack beforehand. This preemptive approach helps curb excessive hunger and reduces the temptation to indulge in carb-heavy appetizers or desserts. When you arrive at the restaurant already satiated, you are better equipped to make mindful, keto-compliant choices.

Meal timing can also be adjusted when dining out. If you practice intermittent fasting, plan your eating window around your restaurant visit. This coordination allows you to enjoy your meal without breaking your fast prematurely or feeling pressured to eat when you're not hungry.

Finally, cultivate a sense of joy and gratitude in your dining experiences. Celebrating food as a source of nourishment and pleasure, rather than restriction, fosters a positive relationship with eating that fuels your ketogenic journey. Remember, each meal out is an opportunity to practice mindfulness, make empowered choices, and enjoy the company of others without compromising your health goals.

In sum, dining out on keto is less about sacrifice and more about savvy strategy and self-respect. With preparation, clear communication, smart ordering, and an assertive mindset, you can navigate any menu with confidence. Your ketogenic lifestyle remains intact, your taste buds delighted, and your health goals steadily progressing — all while enjoying the richness of life's social and culinary experiences.

Knowing how to handle unexpected situations is also part of mastering dining out on keto. Sometimes menus won't list all ingredients, or the kitchen may not be fully aware of your needs. In those moments, trust your instincts and opt for the simplest dishes—plain grilled proteins and steamed vegetables are often safe bets. Don't hesitate to politely decline complicated or "chef's special" items if they don't fit your macros. Your health comes first, and it's perfectly acceptable to make choices that prioritize your well-being over convenience or curiosity.

Social pressure can be another challenge. Friends and family may question your choices or encourage you to "just have a bite" of something off-plan. Being prepared with a clear explanation—focused on your commitment to health and how you feel better following keto—helps deflect judgment and keeps you accountable. You might even inspire curiosity or respect when others see the positive effects of your lifestyle.

When it comes to desserts at restaurants, this can often be the trickiest part of dining out keto. Most classic desserts are sugar bombs, but some places might offer cheese plates, berries with cream, or dark chocolate options that align better with your diet. Don't be shy about asking if the kitchen can create a special keto-friendly dessert or simply enjoy a cup of coffee or herbal tea after your meal. Many keto practitioners find that their cravings for sweets diminish over time, making dessert less of a temptation and more of a mindful treat.

In some cases, bringing your own keto-friendly snacks or desserts to social gatherings can be a lifesaver. This not only ensures you have something delicious and compliant to enjoy but also shares the gift of keto hospitality with others, potentially sparking new interest and support within your circle.

One practical hack for frequent diners is to build a list of favorite restaurants with keto-friendly menus or adaptable dishes. Keep notes on what you order and what works well so that when plans arise, you can confidently choose from known options. This preparation reduces stress and makes keto dining feel second nature rather than a constant battle.

Ultimately, dining out successfully on keto is a blend of preparation, communication, assertiveness, and self-trust. Each meal away from home is an opportunity to reinforce your commitment, celebrate nourishing food, and enjoy the rich variety of flavors available around the world. With these tools and mindset, you turn what might seem like a restriction into a source of empowerment and enjoyment, making your ketogenic lifestyle not just sustainable but truly enjoyable no matter where life takes you.

CHAPTER 23 — KETO MEAL PLANNING AND PREPPING

In the journey of adopting a ketogenic lifestyle, one of the most pivotal elements to ensuring long-term success is mastering the art of meal planning and prepping. This chapter dives deep into the strategies that will transform your keto experience from chaotic and stressful to organized and effortless. When you have a clear, structured plan in place, the daily challenges of choosing the right foods, resisting temptations, and managing your time dissolve, making room for consistent progress and true freedom within your diet.

At the heart of effective keto meal planning is the commitment to clarity and foresight. It's easy to feel overwhelmed by the multitude of choices or to find yourself scrambling for a quick bite that may not align with your macronutrient goals. Having a well-thought-out weekly meal calendar puts an end to this uncertainty. When you know exactly what you will eat each day, the temptation to stray decreases drastically, and your grocery shopping becomes purposeful and efficient. This calendar acts as your roadmap, highlighting breakfast, lunch, dinner, and even snack options that fit perfectly within your keto framework, tailored to your preferences, lifestyle, and goals.

Meal prepping takes this planning a step further. By dedicating time to prepare ingredients or entire meals ahead of time, you unlock a treasure trove of convenience that fuels your ketogenic success. The busy days that once felt like obstacles now become manageable because your meals are ready to go, freeing you from last-minute decisions that often lead to carb-heavy pitfalls. Prepping doesn't mean you need to cook every meal in advance but rather organize components like chopped vegetables, cooked proteins, sauces, or even full dishes that can be quickly assembled or reheated. This strategy not only saves time but preserves your energy for more important pursuits.

One of the most efficient techniques within meal prepping is batch cooking. This approach lets you prepare several servings of a particular dish in one go, allowing you to store leftovers for multiple days or freeze portions for later use. Imagine spending an afternoon slow-cooking a savory beef stew, roasting a tray of seasoned vegetables, or baking a casserole that can sustain your lunches and dinners for the upcoming week. Not only does this reduce the stress of daily cooking, but it also helps control portion sizes and nutritional balance, key factors in maintaining ketosis.

In the modern keto kitchen, appliances like slow cookers, pressure cookers, and sheet pans become invaluable allies. These tools make cooking effortless, often requiring minimal hands-on time while delivering rich, flavorful meals. Slow cookers, for instance, allow you to combine ingredients and set them to cook while you attend to other tasks, returning to a warm, ready-to-eat meal. Pressure cookers speed up cooking times without sacrificing texture or taste, ideal for busy individuals who still crave home-cooked meals. Sheet pan recipes are especially convenient because they involve tossing ingredients on a single pan and baking, simplifying both preparation and cleanup.

A well-designed meal plan isn't complete without a thoughtfully curated grocery list. This list, based on your weekly menu, ensures you purchase only what you need, cutting down on food waste and keeping your pantry stocked with keto staples. It includes high-quality fats like olive oil, coconut oil, and butter; a variety of proteins such as grass-fed beef, free-range chicken, and wild-caught fish; and a colorful array of low-carb vegetables to keep your plate vibrant and nutrient-dense. Having this list in hand before shopping trips saves time and minimizes impulse buys, which can derail your progress.

Proper storage and food handling are equally critical components of meal prepping. Learning the best ways to store prepped ingredients and cooked meals preserves freshness, flavor, and nutritional value. Whether you're refrigerating chopped vegetables in airtight containers or freezing individual portions in meal-sized bags, knowing how to maintain quality ensures you enjoy your food as intended. Reheating techniques matter too — gentle warming prevents drying out or overcooking, keeping textures appealing and appetites satisfied.

Above all, consistency reigns supreme in keto meal planning and prepping. By taking control of your food environment, you reduce the likelihood of reaching for carb-laden snacks or skipping meals altogether. With your kitchen stocked, your meals prepared, and a plan guiding your days, the ketogenic lifestyle becomes not a burden but a seamless part of your routine. Each meal becomes an opportunity to nourish your body, support your metabolism, and deepen your commitment to health.

As you embark on refining your meal planning and prepping skills, remember that flexibility is your friend. Life is dynamic, and while having a plan is empowering, being adaptable allows you to respond to social events, unexpected schedule changes, or sudden cravings without guilt. Over time, this balance of structure and freedom builds resilience, making ketosis sustainable and enjoyable for the long haul.

This chapter also includes sample meal plans tailored for different levels of experience and caloric needs, illustrating how to balance fats, proteins, and carbohydrates while keeping meals exciting. From simple breakfasts that you can prep in bulk to elaborate dinners that can be batched and frozen, these examples provide a blueprint to customize and expand upon according to your tastes.

By integrating these strategies, your ketogenic journey becomes less about daily survival and more about thriving. Meal planning and prepping are not just chores but powerful tools that unlock the full potential of keto living, helping you reach your goals with confidence and ease. Whether you're just starting or seeking to refine your routine, this chapter equips you with the knowledge and motivation to take control of your nutrition and enjoy the many rewards of the ketogenic lifestyle.

The beauty of meal planning and prepping within a ketogenic framework lies not only in the physical benefits but also in the psychological peace it brings. When your meals are thoughtfully prepared ahead of time, the mental burden of decision fatigue lightens. You no longer find yourself standing in front of an open fridge, overwhelmed by choices, or worse, surrendering to convenience foods that threaten your ketosis. Instead, you feel empowered—armed with a clear plan and delicious, ready-to-eat options that honor your health goals.

Meal prepping also fosters creativity in the kitchen. When you allocate time to prepare meals in bulk, you can experiment with flavors and ingredients that may seem daunting during a rushed weekday evening. Slow-roasted herbs, infused oils, spice blends, and layered textures become part of your culinary toolkit, elevating simple dishes into gourmet experiences. This creative engagement not only keeps your meals interesting but deepens your connection to your food, turning nourishment into an act of joy rather than obligation.

Another key advantage is how meal prepping supports portion control. When you prepare meals in advance, you can measure and portion your ingredients precisely, ensuring each plate fits within your macro goals. This discipline helps prevent overeating or undereating, both of which can derail progress. Pre-portioning also saves time when hunger strikes, as you can grab a perfectly sized meal without the need to prepare or guess portions on the fly.

Embracing meal planning means reducing food waste as well. By buying only what your weekly menu requires and using leftovers creatively, you minimize the environmental and financial cost of discarded food. For example, last night's roast chicken can be transformed into a vibrant keto chicken salad or incorporated into an omelette the next morning. This resourcefulness stretches your grocery dollars and keeps your meals fresh and exciting.

The intersection of meal prepping and intermittent fasting also deserves mention. Many keto practitioners find that prepping nutrient-dense meals ahead of their eating windows supports both satiety and convenience. Having ready-made meals aligns seamlessly with the timing and structure of fasting protocols, making adherence simpler and more enjoyable. For those experimenting with time-restricted eating or longer fasts, knowing that a wholesome, ketogenic meal awaits can ease the transition back to eating and reinforce positive habits.

In the realm of keto meal planning, shopping smartly is equally crucial. Opt for seasonal, organic produce when possible, to maximize nutrients and flavor. Prioritize whole, unprocessed foods over packaged alternatives to avoid hidden carbs, additives, and preservatives. Building relationships with local farmers or specialty markets can provide access to fresh, high-quality ingredients that elevate your dishes. Equally, understanding labels and ingredient lists guards against sneaky carbs and sugars that can sneak into seemingly keto-friendly products.

Meal prepping also paves the way for mindful eating. With the effort and care invested in your meals, you are more likely to slow down and savor each bite, tuning into hunger and fullness cues. This mindfulness not only enhances digestion but reinforces the intuitive relationship with food that keto encourages, where nourishment is respected, and overeating is less common.

As you become more experienced with keto meal planning, you will naturally develop your signature staples—go-to recipes that satisfy your palate and macros with ease. These staples serve as anchors around which you build variety, ensuring that you never feel stuck or uninspired. Having these favorites on rotation reduces planning time and decision fatigue, allowing more mental bandwidth for other priorities.

While it may seem that meal prepping requires an upfront time investment, this effort pays dividends throughout your week. What might take an hour or two on a Sunday can save countless minutes during hectic mornings and evenings, preventing stress and encouraging consistency. Over time, this rhythm becomes second nature, a comforting ritual that supports your well-being.

Incorporating family or household members into meal planning and prepping can further enhance success. Sharing responsibilities and tastes fosters communal commitment, making the keto lifestyle a shared experience rather than an isolated challenge. It also allows you to explore recipes that appeal to diverse preferences, ensuring everyone enjoys satisfying, nutritious meals without compromise.

This chapter also encourages you to track and adjust. Using food journals, apps, or simple notes helps monitor how different meals affect your energy, mood, and ketosis. This feedback loop enables you to refine your menu, swap out less enjoyable options, and identify new favorites that keep your nutrition aligned with your goals.

Ultimately, mastering keto meal planning and prepping is about cultivating a lifestyle that harmonizes discipline with flexibility, preparation with spontaneity, and health with enjoyment. As you deepen your understanding of your body's needs and your culinary preferences, you build a sustainable foundation for long-term success.

With the right tools, mindset, and recipes, your keto journey becomes less a daily battle and more a celebration of nourishing, flavorful food that fuels your best self. This chapter invites you to embrace meal planning and prepping not as chores but as empowering acts of self-care—cornerstones of your transformation and wellness.

CHAPTER 24 — OVERCOMING PLATEAUS AND SETBACKS

When you embark on a ketogenic journey, you're signing up for a powerful transformation — not a straight path to overnight success, but a rich, deep process of change that involves your body, your mind, and your lifestyle. It's a path filled with progress, breakthroughs, and sometimes plateaus and temporary backsteps. There will come a moment when you find yourself stranded on a weight-loss plateau, when the scale seems to be ignoring your hard work, when your jeans aren't feeling looser, and when you start to question whether you're truly on the right path. That moment, however, is not a failure; it's a very normal, temporary pause in your progress — a sign that your body is making adjustments and that your metabolism is going through its own process of recalibration.

Your body is a remarkable, adaptable machine. As you cut back on carbohydrates and become proficient at using fats for energy, numerous internal mechanisms respond in kind. Your body drops water as its glycogen stores diminish; it starts to release fatty acids into your bloodstream and produce ketones; and it performs a dramatic metabolic shift to align itself with this new way of eating. Naturally, this isn't a straight descent downward on the scale; there are moments when the body temporarily holds fluids, adds muscle, or simply adjusts its metabolic rate in response to reduced calorie intake. Sometimes what feels like a stall isn't a true stall at all — it may be your body adding muscle mass or retaining water — or simply a temporary pause in a much longer trend.

This is where patience and persistence become your greatest allies. Instead of reacting impulsively — cutting back drastically on calories or adding strenuous routines — it's often more helpful to reassess and fine-tune your approach. Begin by looking honestly at your calorie intake. Sometimes we become a little more generous with serving sizes or allow hidden carbohydrates to sneak back into our diet. Small deviations — a handful of almonds here, a few drops of a creamy salad dressing there — can add up quickly and undermine progress without us realizing it. It's worth keeping a food journal, at least temporarily, to illuminate these hidden sources of carbohydrate and calories.

Reducing calorie intake slightly or adding physical activity can sometimes help move you forward. A walk after dinner, a short resistance training session, or swapping a heavy meal for something lighter can make a surprisingly large difference in your progress. Furthermore, extending your fasts — perhaps adding an additional 16-hour or 24-hour fast once or twice a week — can help your body break through a stall by depleting its glycogen and forcing it back into a state of deep ketosis. Nonetheless, these tweaks should be made judiciously and with consideration for your lifestyle, health conditions, and stress levels.

Some plateaus are influenced by factors we often ignore, such as poor sleep, chronic stress, or dehydration. Your body interprets stress — whether physical or psychological — as a potential threat. Elevated stress signals the release of adrenaline and the stress hormone, cortisol. Higher stress and poor sleep can affect your ability to lose weight by causing water retention, interfering with your ability to regulate blood sugar, and dampening the body's ability to efficiently utilize its own fatty stores. Making relaxation, proper rest, and hydration a priority can profoundly affect your progress.

Sleep is a powerful tool for recovery, hormonal balance, and metabolic health. A consistent seven to nine hours of restful sleep each night allow your body to repair muscle, regulate stress responses, and release growth hormones that aid in recovery and renewal. Furthermore, staying adequately hydrated assists in proper metabolic function, assists in the removal of waste products, and prevents fluids from being inappropriately held in tissues. Sometimes simply drinking more water, reducing sodium intake, or adding a small amount of magnesium or potassium can ease a temporary stall and allow progress to resume.

Another consideration during a stall is your consumption of alcohol, dairy, and sweeteners — all of which can affect your progress in subtle ways. Naturally sweetened products, while calorie-free, can sometimes affect cravings and undermine discipline. Certain alcohols, particularly those made from grains or adding sugars, can interrupt ketosis and slow progress. Dairy products — heavy cream, yogurt, and hard cheeses — although low in carbohydrates, can sometimes contribute to a stall due to their calorie density and the effects of dairy proteins on inflammation and water retention. If you find yourself at a persistent plateau, consider reducing or temporarily eliminating these from your diet and reassess their effects.

Your progress is a marathon, not a sprint. It's a journey filled with signals from your body — signals you need to learn to interpret and respond to in a calm, measured, and constructive way. Staying the course, honoring your progress, and trusting the process will allow you to move through plateaus and come out the other side more resilient and more in control of your health.

As you move forward on this path, it's helpful to view plateaus not as roadblocks but as rest stops — points where your body is pausing to reassess and stabilize before making its next descent toward health and wellness. There is a powerful physiology at work here. Your body is designed to maintain homeostasis; it's hardwired to resist dramatic fluctuations in weight and energy stores. So when you lose a significant amount of weight, it's not unusual for your body to temporarily "push back"— slowing your progress and conserving resources. Naturally, this can be frustrating, but it's a normal part of a successful, sustained transformation.

Instead of battling against this process, it's more effective to work with it. Give your body time to adjust; appreciate these plateaus as signals that you're making profound internal change. During this period, it's a perfect opportunity to reassess your goals and routines. Are you honoring your carbohydrate limits? Are you choosing whole, unprocessed foods over convenient, processed alternatives? Are you paying close attention to hidden ingredients — the starch in a creamy soup base, the dextrose in a marinade — that might undermine your progress?

Some people find it helpful at this point to cut back on all sources of sweetening — even non-caloric ones — and simplify their diet. Eating a few well-chosen, simple foods, rich in healthy fats and proteins, can sometimes help the body "reset" and allow progress to move forward once more. Lean cuts of steak, fatty fish, avocado, olive oil, and a handful of non-starchy veggies can form a powerful baseline from which your body can reignite its ability to burn stored fat.

Additionally, consider your activity level and stress reduction techniques. Are you sitting all day, not adding movement to your routine? Small lifestyle tweaks — choosing the stairs over the elevator, adding a short walk after dinner, or trying a gentle resistance training program — can collectively make a huge difference in how your body utilizes its energy and handles stress. Furthermore, relaxation practices — meditation, journaling, deep-breathing exercises — help to lower stress, reducing the production of stress hormones and thereby freeing your body to let go of excess weight.

Some people find it helpful to track their progress in more ways than just the scale. Measuring your waist, hips, and thighs can be a more accurate reflection of fat-loss, particularly if you're adding muscle. A pair of jeans fitting more comfortably, a belt needing a tighter notch, or simply feeling more energetic and less bloated can be powerful indicators that your body is changing in a healthy direction — even when the scale temporarily stalls.

Your progress might be a marathon, not a sprint, but it's a profoundly rewarding journey. The strategies you implement during a plateau — patience, discipline, careful observation — become powerful lifestyle habits that will serve you well long after you reach your goals. Instead of feeling discouraged, you come to appreciate these periods for what they are:

opportunities to reflect, fine-tune, and grow in knowledge and confidence.

In this context, it's helpful to remember your "why"— the deep, powerful motivation that drove you to pursue this path in the first place. Whether it's to reverse a health condition, lose excess weight, improve energy and confidence, or simply feel more comfortable in your own skin — reconnecting with this "why" during plateaus can provide renewal and perseverance.

Your body is not a simple machine; it's a complex, adaptive ecosystem. It responds to signals, stressors, nutrients, and lifestyle factors in sophisticated ways. So when you find yourself temporarily at a standstill, it's not a failure; it's a powerful opportunity to reassess, adjust, and move forward more intelligently and gracefully.

CHAPTER 25 — STAYING MOTIVATED LONG TERM

There's a powerful thread tying together all successful journeys — motivation. It's the spark that starts you off and the deep well you draw from when obstacles arise. Staying motivated on your ketogenic journey isn't about a fleeting feeling; it's about cultivating a mindset, a way of thinking and acting, that guides you forward day after day. It's about honoring your health, honoring your future, and honoring yourself. To stay motivated long term, you need to connect to something greater than momentary temptation. You need to connect to your "why"—your most profound, powerful reasons for choosing this lifestyle in the first place.

Your "why" might be different from someone else's. It might be the ability to chase after your children without feeling fatigued, or it might be a deep health crisis you're battling against and a ketogenic lifestyle is your path back toward health and renewal. Whatever it is, this "why" must reside in your soul, not just in your mind. It should be something you feel in your gut, something that resonates with your greatest desires. Whenever temptation calls, you can return to this "why"—this deep purpose—as your anchor, your North Star, guiding you back toward your goals.

Setting realistic goals is another key component of staying motivated. It's easy to become discouraged if you aim for dramatic change overnight. Instead, break your goals into small, doable milestones. Celebrate each small win — whether it's dropping your first 5 lbs, fitting into jeans you hadn't worn in years, or seeing your energy soar and your health markers improve. Each small triumph is a piece of your future, a brick in the path you're creating for yourself. It's these small, consistent progress points that add up to dramatic transformation over time.

Non-scale victories, in particular, can be a powerful motivational tool. The scale is a blunt, sometimes unreliable instrument for measuring progress. It doesn't reflect reduced inflammation, greater energy, or a newfound ability to keep up with your children or grandkids. It certainly doesn't reflect lowered blood sugar, improved cholesterol, or a dramatic drop in blood pressure — all dramatic health improvements that often come from a ketogenic lifestyle. So it's crucial to celebrate these non-scale victories. Take progress photos, track your energy levels, jot down health indicators from your doctor's visits. The more you appreciate these subtle but powerful signals of progress, the more motivated you'll become to stay the course.

Support groups can be a huge help in maintaining motivation. Surround yourself with people who appreciate and celebrate your progress. Whether you find a community online, connect with a friend, or recruit a family member to do it alongside you, having a support network makes all the difference. There will be tough days — days when temptation feels overwhelming or when progress seems to stall — and having someone who "gets it" can be profoundly validating. Support groups allow you to celebrate milestones together, learn from each other's struggles, and stay motivated through communal encouragement.

Journaling your progress is another powerful tool. There's something about putting your thoughts and achievements into words that makes them more real, more permanent. Keep a health journey notebook where you track your food intake, your physical activity, your progress photos, and your health markers. Write honestly about your struggles, your doubts, and your triumphs. The act of journaling lets you reflect on how far you've come and how much you've grown, adding momentum to carry you forward. Whenever you feel discouraged, you can look back at those pages and realize you're not the person you were when you started — you're stronger, more resilient, and more in control of your choices.

Pairing goals with non-food rewards is another powerful motivational tactic. Naturally, when we celebrate achievements, we often gravitate toward food — a nice dinner, a rich dessert — but this can undermine progress and send mixed signals to your subconscious. Instead, treat yourself to something that nurtures your lifestyle and health — a new pair of jeans, a spa day, a cooking gadget to aid in meal preparation, or a fitness tracker. Small rewards honoring your progress help you stay motivated without derailing you from your goals. Importantly, these rewards become a form of self-care; you're honoring yourself for honoring your health.

Getting back on track quickly after a deviation is a key piece of motivation. There will be days when you eat something you hadn't intended or when you temporarily lose your discipline. That's okay; you're human. The crucial part is how quickly you respond and move forward. Small deviations do not erase all your progress — it's persistent habits over time that produce dramatic change. So instead of letting a small slip spiral into a full-on derailment, learn from it, put it in perspective, and move forward immediately. The faster you do this, the less power temptation has over you.

Your discipline, patience, and growth mindset are what will carry you through the tough days. Staying motivated isn't about feeling excited all the time; it's about honoring your goals even when you're tired, discouraged, or unsure. It's about trusting the process, trusting yourself, and trusting that small, consistent choices add up to dramatic transformation. It's about choosing the future you want over the moment you're in. That discipline transforms a diet into a lifestyle — a permanent, powerful change in the way you nourish your body and care for yourself.

Ultimately, staying motivated comes from honoring yourself and honoring your health. It comes from understanding that you are worth it — worth the effort, the patience, the discipline — to become the person you want to be. The ketogenic lifestyle is not a punishment; it's a powerful tool for renewal and transformation. It's a path back to health, back to confidence, back to energy and happiness. It's a way to take control of your future, instead of letting temptation, health struggles, or poor habits dictate it for you.

Your motivation is a reflection of your deep care for yourself. It's a form of love — choosing health over temptation, choosing discipline over indulgence — that transforms not just your body, but your whole life. It's a powerful journey, filled with small triumphs and big breakthroughs. And it all starts from within — from your resolve, your "why", and your ability to stay the course.

Your motivation is not a straight path; it's a rich and winding journey filled with lessons, revelations, and moments of deep transformation. There will be days when you feel a rush of progress — when you realize your jeans are fitting more loosely, your energy is soaring, and your health markers are improving — and there will be days when it feels like you're battling against temptation, stress, and overwhelm. The key is understanding that this range of experiences is all part of the process. It's not a sign of failure; it's a sign you're growing, evolving, and strengthening your resolve.

One powerful way to stay motivated is to view these fluctuations through a growth mindset. Instead of seeing struggles or plateaus as roadblocks, view them as stepping stones — opportunities to learn more about yourself, about your triggers, and about what strategies help you stay strong. Did you find yourself slipping after a particularly hectic day at work or a social gathering filled with temptation? That's not a failure; it's valuable information. It highlights a vulnerable spot in your routine — a place you can fortify in the future by planning ahead, preparing a fallback meal, or simply employing stress-reduction techniques.

Your motivation deepens when you realize you're not powerless in the face of temptation; you're adaptable and resilient. The more you navigate these moments successfully, the more confidence you develop in your ability to conquer future obstacles. That confidence — that deep "I've gotten through hard things before; I can do it again"— is a powerful motivational force.

This lifestyle isn't about perfection; it's about progress. There will be slips and struggles, but what matters most is your ability to learn from them and move forward. Small deviations, when dealt with promptly and compassionately, become a minor blip in your overall trajectory instead of a dramatic reversal. Your ability to respond gracefully — without shame, without all-or-none thinking — is a key piece of staying motivated and staying the course.

Another tactic to keep motivation alive is to regularly reconnect with your "why." Take time each day, or at least each week, to reflect on what you're trying to achieve and why it matters to you. Visualize your future — not just your physical appearance, but how you will feel, how you will move through the world, how much more energy you will have, and how much more confidence you will exude. Picture yourself playing with your children without tiring, wearing the clothes you love without discomfort, or simply waking up in the morning feeling rested, clearheaded, and excited about the day.

This kind of visualization has a powerful motivational effect because it makes your future feel real and achievable. It transforms your goals from an abstract wish into a vivid, desirable future you're already creating. Whenever temptation strikes or motivation falters, you can close your eyes and reconnect with this future, letting it pull you forward and illuminate your choices in the present.

Your surroundings can profoundly affect motivation as well. If your home is filled with temptation — chips in the cupboard, cookies on the counter — you're making it hard for yourself to stay on track. Take the time to clear out foods that undermine you and stock your kitchen with ingredients that align with your goals. Display healthy snacks at the ready — hard-boiled eggs, cut-up veggies, small handfuls of almonds — and put temptation out of view. Your environment should reflect your goals and support your choices, not undermine them.

This extends to your social surroundings, too. If you have friends or relatives who dismiss or undermine your choices, it may be helpful to limit your time with them or to set clear boundaries about what you will and will not eat when you're together. Surround yourself instead with people who celebrate your progress, who appreciate your discipline, and who want to see you become your best self. Support is a powerful motivational tool; it's hard to stay motivated when you're surrounded by negativity, but when you're supported and encouraged, motivation comes much more naturally.

Your routines and habits form the foundation of motivation. Small, daily habits — choosing a ketogenic meal, drinking plenty of water, going for a walk — become powerful signals to your brain and body that you're a person who is committed to health. Each time you follow through, you're casting a vote for the person you want to become. It's a form of behavioral momentum; the more you do it, the more automatic it becomes. At first, you may need discipline and willpower to stay on track, but over time these choices become effortless, woven into your lifestyle and your sense of self.

Some find it helpful to track progress daily — marking off each day you stayed ketogenic, noting physical activity, or journaling about your choices. There's a motivational rush from seeing a string of days adding up, a literal "chain" of discipline that you're proud not to break. There are many habit tracker apps and calendars available to help you visualize this progress and celebrate your consistency.

Your motivation can also be sustained by education — by deepening your understanding of the ketogenic lifestyle and the mechanisms that make it effective. The more you appreciate how profoundly a low carbohydrate diet can affect your physiology — reducing insulin resistance, improving metabolic health, quelling inflammation — the more you realize you're not making a small change; you're making a dramatic, health-changing transformation. That knowledge anchors you; it converts temptation into a lesser consideration, a momentary feeling, not a powerful force. Your choices become purposeful and informed.

This understanding also helps you appreciate the adaptability of your body. Your ability to produce ketones for energy, to become a "fat burner" instead of a "sugar burner"—this is a dramatic metabolic shift. It signals a deep healing process; you're turning back years of poor health and poor habits. Whenever you feel discouraged, you can remember that your body is designed to do this; it wants to heal and flourish under the right conditions. Your motivation, then, is a form of collaboration with your physiology; you're simply providing the conditions for health to manifest.

Ultimately, motivation comes from honoring your future self — the person you're becoming. It comes from choosing not what feels easy in the moment, but what will serve you in the long term. It's a form of maturity, a deep understanding that you're not a slave to your impulses; you're a person with goals, with discipline, and with the ability to shape your own future. Each meal, each choice, each day is a step forward on this path.

As you progress, motivation transforms from a feeling you chase into a state you inhabit. It permeates your routines, your decisions, your lifestyle. It's not something you need to find; it's something you become. Your discipline, your choices, and your progress all reflect this deep transformation.

Your motivation is a powerful force — not because it's perfect or effortless, but because it's sustained by something greater than momentary temptation. It's sustained by your values, your goals, and your deep understanding of what you're creating in your life. It's a reflection of your ability to grow, to adapt, and to conquer whatever stands in your path.

CHAPTER 26 — WORKOUT AND KETO SYNERGY

There's a powerful synergy that emerges when you combine a well-formulated ketogenic diet with a thoughtful and purposeful approach to physical activity. It's a synergy that transforms not only your body composition but also your metabolic health, your energy levels, and your ability to perform daily tasks with ease. Inside this rich marriage of diet and movement lies a key to unlocking a powerful transformation — a way to align your physiology and lifestyle in a manner that lets you become the strongest, healthiest, and most vital version of yourself.

When you first embark on a ketogenic diet, your body undergoes a dramatic metabolic shift. It starts to move away from a reliance on glucose and carbohydrates for energy and instead starts to produce and utilize ketones — small, energy-dense molecules made from fatty acids — to power its cells. At first, this can be a challenging period of adaptation. Your muscles, your liver, and your brain need time to learn how to efficiently use this new form of energy. It's not unusual during the first few weeks to feel sluggish, weak, or less explosive in your physical movements. Your body is in a state of metabolic reprogramming, dialing back its dependence on an abundance of glucose and turning instead toward a more stable and sustained energy base.

Once you move through this adaptation period and become fully "fat-adaptation proficient"— a state where your body efficiently converts fatty acids into ketones and utilizes them for energy — a dramatic change occurs. Your ability to perform sustained, low to medium-intensity activity increases. Hiking, jogging, cycling, and other forms of movement that predominantly rely on the aerobic energy systems become more effortless. The slow, steady release of energy from fatty acid oxidation lets you keep going without the dramatic drops in energy that you may have previously experienced when your body was tied to a carbohydrate-dependent metabolism.

Strength training and resistance exercise have a unique role to play in this context. Lifting weights, body-weight resistance, or employing resistance bands signals your body to maintain and grow muscle mass, even while you are in a calorie deficit. Naturally, a well-formulated ketogenic diet already assists in preserving muscle by reducing the catabolic effects of stress and by offering a rich supply of proteins and essential fatty acids. But adding resistance training compounds these benefits. It signals to your body that muscle is a key and necessary component of your physiology — not something it can break down for energy. Furthermore, adding muscle mass increases your resting metabolic rate, helping you burn more calories and become more efficient at using energy.

Some people find their explosive, high-intensity movements — sprints, heavy power lifting, explosive Olympic lifts — suffer temporarily during the initial adaptation. That's because these activities predominantly rely on a phosphocreatine and glycolytic energy system, which normally depends on a ready supply of glucose. During adaptation, when muscle glycogen drops and the body is shifting its metabolic machinery toward fats and ketones, explosive power can diminish temporarily. But this is a temporary phenomenon. Once adaptation is complete and your body settles into its new metabolic baseline, many find their explosive capabilities return, often alongside a dramatic improvement in their ability to perform sustained activity without tiring quickly.

Your diet plays a key role in shaping this process. Consuming a well-formulated ketogenic diet — rich in healthy fats, filled with sources of complete proteins, and kept low in carbohydrate — provides a strong foundation for physical activity and recovery. It dampens the production of reactive oxygen species and chronic inflammation, letting your muscles repair more efficiently after a tough workout. It stabilises your energy, preventing dramatic drops in blood sugar and letting you perform at a more consistent level. Furthermore, a ketogenic diet assists in conserving muscle mass during calorie deficits — something many people find challenging under a conventional diet — and this, in turn, helps to maintain metabolic health and physical functionality.

Your choice of activity should reflect your goals and preferences. If you prefer low-impact movement, walking and cycling align nicely with a ketogenic physiology. If you enjoy resistance training, a regimen of heavy compound movements — squats, deadlifts, pull-ups — performed a few times per week can be profoundly effective. Yoga, kettlebells, and body-weight circuits are all viable methods for strengthening and conditioning your body while honoring its unique energy systems. The key is to match your activity to your diet, your goals, and your lifestyle in a way that feels sustainable and enjoyable.

Pairing diet and movement this way lets you maximize the benefits of both. The ketogenic diet provides a stable, adaptable energy base, and physical activity signals your body to grow strong and resilient. It's a powerful combination — a synergy — that transforms you from the inside out. Your muscles become more efficient at using fatty acids; your mitochondria become more numerous and more effective; your ability to perform physical tasks, from a simple walk in the park to a challenging resistance training session, expands. The result is a dramatic improvement in health, body composition, energy, and a deep, enduring feeling of physical well-being.

Ultimately, this synergy between diet and movement underscores a key principle of human physiology: we are designed to move, and we are designed to use a range of energy sources efficiently. The ketogenic diet simply provides the metabolic framework to maximize these capabilities. With patience, persistence, and a willingness to learn, you can align your diet and your activity to become a strong, adaptable, and healthy person — someone who finds movement a natural expression of their health and who draws energy effortlessly from their own body's stores.

Your transformation lies not in choosing between diet or exercise, but in understanding how profoundly the two are connected. The ketogenic diet is not just a tool for weight control — it's a powerful ally for physical performance. Pair it with a movement regimen tailored to your goals and preferences, and you will find yourself unlocking a level of health, fitness, and energy you may have thought were unreachable. Whatever your starting point, this combination holds the potential to carry you forward into a future filled with vitality, strength, and enduring well-being.

As you progress further into your ketogenic journey and become more proficient at using fatty acids and ketones for energy, something remarkable starts to happen at the cellular level. The number and density of your mitochondria — the tiny powerhouses within your cells — increase in a process called mitochondrial biogenesis. This expansion means you have more "engines" available to produce energy efficiently and more raw power to draw upon when you need it.

This mitochondrial adaptation underpins much of the enhanced physical performance that people report after a period of deep ketogenic adaptation. Your muscles become not just strong but metabolically flexible — able to generate energy from both fatty acids and, when required, from the small amount of glucose you produce internally. Your body is no longer a fragile machine that falters under stress; instead, it evolves into a robust, adaptable, and enduring apparatus — perfect for sustained physical activity.

This adaptability is particularly useful during medium-intensity efforts — jogging, rowing, cycling at a comfortable but challenging pace — where the predominant energy demand can be fully supported by fatty acid oxidation and ketone utilization. The result is a dramatic reduction in the phenomenon known as "bonking"— a dramatic drop in energy — because your body is no longer limited by a small pool of muscle glycogen. Instead, it has a vast reserve of energy in its own body-fat stores — a reserve you can tap into nearly endlessly.

Meanwhile, resistance training signals your body to retain and grow muscle, adding a protective layer of metabolic health. The more muscle you have, the more efficiently you dispose of glucose, and the less likely you are to develop disorders related to poor glucose regulation. Furthermore, muscle is a metabolically-active tissue; it plays a key role in resting energy expenditure and the disposal of excess nutrients. So the more muscle you retain or develop through resistance training, the greater your ability to maintain a healthy body composition and metabolic profile.

Some people find it helpful to match their training to their diet. For example, medium- or lower-intensity sessions — jogging, yoga, cycling — align nicely with a ketogenic physiology. Higher-intensity sessions — heavy lifting, sprint intervals — may require careful consideration. Some people find adding a small amount of carbohydrate (such as 20-30 grams from a whole food source) immediately after a heavy training session assists in recovery without derailing their ketogenic state. Others find their performance is unaffected once fully adapted, reflecting the remarkable ability of the body to produce its own glucose through a process called gluconeogenesis. Whatever your approach, understanding these mechanisms lets you personalize your diet and training to maximize benefits and minimize drawbacks.

Hydration and electrolyte balance become especially important in this context. As your body drops excess water during the initial phases of a ketogenic diet — a phenomenon called natriuresis — sodium, potassium, and magnesium can become temporarily depleted. Replenish these strategically — adding a bit more sodium to your diet, consuming foods rich in potassium and magnesium, or using a supplement if necessary — and you will find your physical performance and recovery improving. Staying adequately hydrated also assists in delivering nutrients to muscles and removing waste products — a key consideration during strenuous activity — and prevents muscle cramps, weakness, and poor recovery.

Sleep, stress, and recovery practices all profoundly affect your ability to perform and progress. A ketogenic diet typically stabilises energy and reduces fluctuations in blood sugar, which can translate into more restful sleep and a greater ability to handle stress. Nevertheless, honoring your body's need for recovery — honoring rest days, employing relaxation techniques, and reducing stress through lifestyle practices — is a key component of sustained progress. Without proper recovery, even the best diet and training will produce sub-optimal results.

This highlights an important principle: diet and movement are not separate components; they form a unified whole. Your physiology responds to signals from your diet, your activity, your rest, and your stress all at once. The more you align these signals — a diet that supports your energy production, activity that stimulates desirable adaptation, rest that allows for recovery, and stress reduction strategies that keep your nervous system from becoming chronically over-active — the more dramatic and lasting your transformation will be.

This synergy extends to your psychology as well. The discipline required to follow a ketogenic diet, to pursue physical activity consistently, and to manage stress effectively instills a powerful sense of control and confidence in your ability to affect your own health and future. There is a deep satisfaction in honoring your body's signals and meeting its needs in a way that produces measurable progress. The result is not just physical transformation, but a newfound resiliency — a ability to face stress and challenge, whether physical or psychological, from a place of stability and confidence.

Your body evolves in response to the signals you send it. Each meal, each training session, each moment of rest, and each decision to pursue health instead of temptation feeds into a powerful, ongoing process of transformation. The synergy of a ketogenic diet and physical activity lets you take control of this process, turning it into a powerful upward spiral — a path toward greater health, greater fitness, and greater happiness.

Some find this journey profoundly transformational, not just physically but mentally and emotionally. It instills a deep understanding of the body's ability to heal, adapt, and grow. It dismantles misconceptions about weakness and limitation and reveals a hidden potential for human health and performance. It shows you that your physiology is not fixed or dictated by your genes or your past — it is a flexible, adaptable, and responsive system that evolves in direct relation to your choices.

This view transforms lifestyle choices from something restrictive into something profoundly empowering. Eating a ketogenic diet and honoring your body's need for movement and recovery become not sacrifices but choices made in service of a greater, more vivid, more energetic future. Your muscles grow strong, your energy stabilises, your mind clears, and your confidence deepens — reflecting a deep, permanent change from the inside out.

CHAPTER 27 — STAYING KETO DURING HOLIDAYS AND EVENTS

The holiday season and special events can be a wonderful time to connect, celebrate, and appreciate all we have in our lives. It's a time filled with rich food, indulgences, and traditions — a time when many find it challenging to stay true to their health goals. But staying ketogenic during holidays and events isn't about missing out; it's about honoring your choices, your health, and your future. It's a powerful affirmation that this lifestyle isn't a temporary diet — it's a permanent, empowering way to live.

Picture a festive dinner table adorned with a rich roast, crispy-skinned chicken, savory cheeses, and a colorful array of low-starchy veggies tossed in herbs and rich butter. The scene is a perfect embodiment of indulgence and satisfaction — without straying from the path you chose. There is a deep peace in honoring your health while participating fully in traditions and ceremonies alongside those you love.

Walking into a holiday dinner or a festive gathering with confidence starts long before you lift your first glass or plate. It starts with a powerful mindset — a deep understanding that you're not depriving yourself, you're honoring yourself. That resolve lets you appreciate a well-cooked piece of steak or a creamy avocado dip just as much as a rich piece of pie — without feeling left out. It lets you celebrate without adding needless carbohydrates back into your diet. It lets you show up fully, without temptation ruling your choices.

One effective strategy to stay true to your lifestyle is to bring a ketogenic dish to a potluck or dinner party. That guarantees you will have something you can eat and enjoy without feeling deprived or stranded in a food environment designed for a very different diet. It could be a creamy cauliflower casserole, a rich spinach and artichoke dip, or a savory plate of crispy-skinned chicken thighs. Whatever you bring, it will not only nourish you, it will show your friends and family that ketogenic food can be indulgent and satisfying.

As you navigate a festive table filled with temptation, remember you have choices. Meats, cheeses, and low-starchy veggies are all fair game. There is something profoundly empowering in choosing foods that align with your goals — honoring not just your taste buds, but your health and future. And when you sip on a sparkling water instead of alcohol or soda, you cut needless calories and carbohydrates without missing a moment of the celebration. That small choice adds up, keeping you firmly in control.

Some people find it helpful to prepare a few phrases to gracefully say "no" when well-meaning friends and relatives press food upon them. A simple, "Thank you, everything looks wonderful, but I'm staying true to my health goals today" or "I appreciate it, but I'm honoring my diet right now" lets you celebrate without causing a scene. It lets you navigate social pressure gracefully and assert your choices with confidence.

This process underscores a powerful shift — you realize you're not a victim of temptation; you're a person making deliberate choices about your health. The more you practice honoring those choices in challenging situations, the more momentum you gain. Each holiday dinner, birthday party, or special event you navigate successfully strengthens your resolve and makes the next one even easier. Your lifestyle becomes less about resistance and more about abundance — a rich array of foods and traditions you can enjoy without straying from your path.

Maintaining discipline during holidays transforms your view of this lifestyle. It shows you that you're not missing a thing — you're gaining health, confidence, and a future filled with opportunity. It highlights a powerful truth: when you align your choices with your goals and values, there's a deep peace and satisfaction that comes from honoring yourself.

Your discipline grows into a form of freedom. The temptation to revert back to old habits lessens, and your confidence strengthens. Your ability to say "yes" to health and "no" to temptation evolves into a powerful affirmation — a deep understanding that this isn't a restrictive diet; it's a rich lifestyle filled with choices that align with your highest goals.

With proper strategies and a strong resolve, you can enjoy all your special moments — holidays, parties, and events — while honoring your health goals. The rich foods you bring, the choices you make, and the confidence you carry reflect a deep transformation. It's a transformation not just of your body, but of your mind and spirit — a transformation that lets you celebrate fully without losing track of where you're headed. So when the next invitation comes, you can respond with confidence, peace, and a deep understanding that you're not missing a thing — you're gaining a future filled with health, happiness, and freedom.

Your future is not a restrictive path; it's a rich, abundant journey filled with delicious food, deep friendships, and a newfound confidence in who you are and what you want. The discipline you practice during holidays and events ripples into all areas of your life — strengthening your ability to resist temptation, pursue goals, and stay true to your highest intentions. It reflects a deep honoring of your health and happiness, a recognition that your choices matter profoundly, not just for your physical well-being but for your future, your relationships, and your ability to show up in the world as your best self.

This discipline evolves into a form of liberation. The moment you realize you're not powerless in the face of temptation — that you can enjoy a rich meal, appreciate a toast with friends, and celebrate without regret — you become free from the cycle of guilt and shame that often accompanies holiday indulgences. Your choices become empowering instead of restrictive, affirming instead of denying.

It's a powerful feeling when you sit back at a festive table, surrounded by those you care about, and know you're honoring your goals while honoring your relationships. There's a deep peace in choosing a plate filled with savory proteins, rich cheeses, and crispy veggies tossed in aromatic herbs and butter — food that makes you feel strong, clear, and in control — instead of yielding to temptation and feeling regret afterwards. It's this peace, this deep satisfaction, that makes the lifestyle sustainable in the long term.

Your ability to stay true to yourself during holidays and events is a reflection of your growing maturity and resolve. It signals to you and everyone around you that you're not someone who drops their goals when temptation strikes; you're someone who stands firm, gracefully, without feeling deprived. It shows a deep understanding that choosing health over momentary indulgences isn't a punishment — it's a powerful affirmation of your future.

Your choices become a form of quiet leadership. Without preaching or making a scene, you become an example for those around you — a person who finds peace and happiness without following the herd. Your discipline, your ability to stay true to your goals, may inspire a friend or a family member to reassess their own choices. It may spark conversations about health, about lifestyle, about honoring oneself in a world that often pushes indulgence over discipline. Your resolve can become a ripple — spreading a culture of health and consideration — far beyond your own plate.

Ultimately, staying ketogenic during holidays and events is not about missing the pleasures of life; it's about choosing a different path to happiness — a path filled with rich food, deep connection, and a clear conscience. It's about honoring your goals and honoring yourself, honoring a future filled with health and opportunity. It's a powerful affirmation that you're not a slave to temptation; you're a master of your choices.

So as you move forward, remember this: you are not powerless. The holidays, the events, the social pressures — all these are a part of life. But you have the ability to navigate them gracefully and successfully. Your discipline will become your greatest asset, a tool you can apply in all aspects of your future.

Your choices today will shape your health, your happiness, and your future. So celebrate with confidence. Celebrate in a way that brings you closer to your goals. Celebrate your ability to conquer temptation and to stay true to yourself. Your future depends on it — and you're more than up to the challenge.

CHAPTER 28 — FINAL PUSH TO TRANSFORMATION

As you enter this final stretch of your 30-Day transformation, there's a powerful momentum at your back — a forward rush — a feeling that you're not the person you were when you first started this journey. The choices you made, the discipline you maintained, and the patience you cultivated have gotten you here, to a place where your body, your mind, and your habits are all aligning in service of your health and your future. It's a remarkable moment — a moment when you realize you have crossed from trial into transformation — from attempting something new into fully owning it.

Your body is no longer unsure about this way of eating; it has become proficient at burning its own fat for energy, instead of always needing a rush of carbohydrates. The metabolic machinery within you — your liver, your muscle cells, your mitochondria — all have made dramatic and permanent adjustments to this new lifestyle. The result is a feeling of sustained energy, mental clarity, and physical stability. There are no more dramatic drops in blood sugar, no more cravings ruling your choices; you have become a powerful, adaptable, and purposeful person who is not a slave to food signals but a master of their own physiology.

This final push is a perfect time to reassess your goals. Look back to where you were when you started — how much you weighed, how you felt in your body, what your health markers were, and most of all, where your mind was. Take a moment to appreciate just how far you have come. Whether you have shed unwanted pounds, reduced your cravings, improved your energy, or lowered health risks, you have made dramatic progress. Your discipline has blossomed into something much more: it has become a permanent part of who you are.

Activity, diet, and mindset all come together at this moment to produce dramatic results. Your muscles respond differently to physical activity now; your body converts fatty acids to energy more efficiently; and your mental resolve has grown in stride with your physical transformation. Your choices at the grocery store, at restaurants, and in your own home reflect a newfound confidence. Your plate no longer resembles the diet of someone battling temptation; it reflects a person who is in control — someone who finds deep satisfaction in choosing foods that nourish and heal.

Some people consider extending their 30-Day plan or making it permanent — and this is a powerful consideration. It signals a dramatic shift in thinking. It shows you are not counting days toward a temporary diet; you are framing this lifestyle as a permanent way forward. The question then becomes not "How much longer can I keep this up?" but "How much more can I achieve?" It highlights the power of momentum. Whatever progress you made in 30 days, imagine what you can do in 60, in 90, or in a year. The discipline you cultivated during this initial period is a strong foundation upon which you can pursue future goals — greater fitness, improved health, a more energetic lifestyle — whatever you choose to pursue.

This chapter guides you through this decision and its implications. Staying the course means honoring routines that have gotten you this far — choosing foods that nourish you, honoring your body's signals of hunger and satiety, and honoring movement as a key to physical health and metabolic adaptability. It also means protecting this progress from backsliding. Small deviations from your diet are a normal part of life — a special meal on a holiday, a dinner with friends — but the discipline you have cultivated lets you navigate those deviations gracefully and without guilt. It lets you appreciate indulgences without losing momentum.

This is a powerful moment, a turning point. Your discipline, patience, and adaptability have gotten you this far. The choices you made — day after day — have made all the difference. The hard days, the doubts, the cravings, the plateaus — you overcame them because you kept going. That perseverance has opened a new path forward. It has transformed not just your body but your mind and your soul. It has shown you a deep well of resolve within yourself — a resolve you can apply to future goals, health-related or not.

Your transformation is not just physical; it's a renewal of your whole self. The person you are now — stronger, more energetic, more disciplined — is the person who will carry you forward into whatever future you wish to create. The discipline you have cultivated will serve you in all aspects of your life, from career goals to relationships to hobbies. The patience you have demonstrated will help you navigate obstacles and disappointments without losing momentum. The adaptability you have mastered will allow you to respond gracefully to whatever comes your way.

As you appreciate this transformation, take a moment to celebrate how much you have grown. Acknowledge the hard choices you made and the sacrifices you overcame. See this not as the end of a diet, but the beginning of a lifestyle — a powerful, purposeful lifestyle — a future filled with health, confidence, and possibilities you hadn't believed were within reach. Your 30-Day transformation is not a finishing line; it's a starting gate. The greatest chapters of your story are yet to be written.

Your transformation has opened a door — a powerful, permanent change — that you can now step through with confidence and resolve. The discipline you cultivated over these past 30 days has become a deep part of you; it has been woven into your routines, your choices, your view of yourself and what you're capable of. It's no longer a temporary discipline — it's a permanent lifestyle, a way of honoring your health and your future.

As you move forward from this milestone, you carry with you not just a thinner body or a clearer mind, but a newfound ability to conquer obstacles and pursue goals that once seemed unreachable. Your discipline has become a tool — a powerful, adaptable tool — that you can apply in countless ways. Want to pursue a physical challenge you previously thought was beyond you — a 5K, a triathlon, or simply a challenging fitness class? Your discipline will carry you there. Want to take a leap in your career or education, learn something new, or conquer a longstanding fear? The resolve you have cultivated will empower you to pursue those goals and more.

Your health journey has demonstrated something profoundly important about human change — it starts from within. It starts from a decision made deep in your soul that you will be more, do more, and become more. It starts from honoring your body's signals and choosing foods and routines that serve you instead of undermine you. It starts from choosing discipline over temptation and patience over instant gratification. The result is transformation — not just a physical change, but a renewal of spirit and character.

Your discipline has a ripple effects, touching not only your own future but the future of those around you. Your children, your friends, your colleagues — all will see your progress and be influenced by it. They may be inspired to make their own health journeys, or to pursue goals that previously seemed unreachable. Your choices become a powerful testimony to the ability of ordinary people to create extraordinary change in their lives.

Your adaptability, patience, and discipline will serve you well, whatever your future holds. If you choose to stay ketogenic, your body will continue to become more proficient at utilizing fatty acids for energy, maintaining muscle mass, and staying strong and healthy. If you pursue a more flexible diet, adding back small amounts of carbohydrates while honoring your body's signals, you will do so from a place of knowledge, confidence, and control — not from a place of temptation or weakness.

Your future health will reflect the choices you make from this day forward. That might mean choosing a rich avocado and grilled steak over a plate of french fries; it might mean honoring your satiety signals instead of ignoring them; it might mean choosing movement over sedentary habits; it might mean honoring rest, stress reduction, and community. All these choices will come more naturally now because you have lived this discipline, you have made it your own, and you have tasted its rewards.

This is the true transformation — not a temporary diet, not a restrictive regimen, but a deep and permanent change in your lifestyle and your relationship with food, movement, and health. It's a renewal of your ability to choose — to respond to your body's signals, to pursue your goals, to become the person you always wanted to be. Whatever your future holds, you carry within you the greatest tool of all — discipline — and with it, there is nothing you cannot achieve.

Your transformation is a powerful story — a story of choosing health over temptation, discipline over indulgence, patience over frustration, and renewal over regret. It's a story you will carry forward into every area of your life. Whenever you face a challenge — a temptation to revert back to old habits, a health hurdle, or a plateaus in progress — you will remember this moment and realize: "I am more than this. I have crossed that bridge already. I know how to navigate this path. I have discipline, patience, adaptability, and resolve. I have transformed myself once; I can do it again and again, if necessary."

Your discipline, patience, and adaptability have gotten you this far — and there is no limit to where you can go from here. The future is yours to shape. Your health is in your hands. Your choices will reflect the person you have become — someone strong, purposeful, and profoundly alive. Embrace this future with confidence, discipline, and a deep, enduring patience. The greatest chapters of your story are yet to come.

CHAPTER 29 — SUSTAINABLE KETO LIVING

There is something profoundly empowering about crossing the 30-Day mark and not looking back. The first few weeks were about adaptation, discipline, and patience. But now you find yourself in a place of deep transformation — not just physically, but mentally and emotionally. The ketogenic lifestyle has permeated all aspects of your health and well-being. It's no longer a restrictive diet you follow in the short term; it's a rich, flexible way of living that evolves alongside you, honoring your goals, preferences, and future health.

Your body has become proficient at using its own stored energy — it converts fatty acids into a powerful and sustained energy called ketones. Your cells, having made this dramatic metabolic shift, are now more adaptable, more resilient, more efficient. Your cravings for carbohydrate-dense foods have diminished, and your taste preferences have shifted toward rich, savory, whole foods — a steak feels more indulgent than a plate of cookies, and a creamy avocado salad is more satisfying than a pile of processed bread. Naturally sweet foods — strawberries, raspberries, a handful of blueberries — become true treats when you do choose to enjoy them.

This is a key moment in your journey. The discipline you cultivated during your first 30 days now evolves into something more effortless. The routines you put in place — meal planning, choosing low carbohydrate ingredients, honoring your hunger signals — are now automatic. It's not a battle against temptation; it's a lifestyle you naturally gravitate toward because you feel and perform your best when you do. Your body has gotten smarter and more adaptable. It can handle a small amount of carbohydrate without spinning back into a metabolic chaos. That's a true indicator of health — flexibility — and it's a hard-won ability.

Some people find it helpful to reassess their carbohydrate intake at this point. If you wish, you can trial adding back small amounts — a serving of sweet potato with dinner once or twice a week, a handful of strawberries in your yogurt, or a piece of dark chocolate after a meal — and observe how you respond. Your body's signals, your energy, your cravings, and your mood will tell you whether this is a comfortable change or a step backward. Sustainable ketogenic living is not a rigid, all-or-none lifestyle; it's a framework you can personalize. It's a way to maximize health while honoring your preferences and goals.

Fitness routines become a powerful counterpart to this diet. The combination of a low carbohydrate lifestyle with physical activity, whether it's resistance training, jogging, cycling, yoga, or simply walking, lets you maintain muscle mass, bone density, and metabolic health. The two together create a synergy — you become a well-fueled, adaptable human, less prone to weakness, injury, and lifestyle-related disease. Your muscles learn to use fatty acids for energy more efficiently; your recovery speeds up; your joints suffer less from inflammation; your mental clarity and focus remain strong.

Your meal plans reflect this maturity. Instead of counting every gram of carbohydrate, you become proficient at choosing whole, rich, low carbohydrate foods. Your plate naturally comprises fatty cuts of meat, wild-caught fish, avocado, olives, non-starchy vegetables tossed in butter or oil, and small amounts of strawberries or raspberries. Herbs and sauces add flavor without adding hidden sugars. Your grocery lists reflect these choices, making meal preparation effortless and enjoyable.

Your future is filled with energy and confidence. There's a peace that comes from trusting your body's signals, honoring its preferences, and choosing foods that align with health, not sickness. The discipline you cultivated during your initial transformation has blossomed into a lifestyle — a way of thinking about food, health, and nourishment. The yo-yo dieting and dramatic swings in energy and weight are gone; you have a stable path forward.

This stability lets you pursue goals outside of diet and health, because you're no longer battling cravings, poor energy, or shame. Your mind is clear; your body feels strong; your confidence grows alongside your discipline. Whether you wish to maintain this lifestyle for years or for a lifetime, you now possess the knowledge and the ability to do so gracefully.

Your transformation signals a permanent change — not a temporary fix — and this is a powerful, hopeful place to be. The future is yours to shape, supported by a lifestyle that nurtures you from the inside out.

As you move forward on this path, you may find that you become a role model for health and discipline in your community — a person whom friends, family, and colleagues look to for guidance and inspiration. Naturally, questions will come up. "How did you do it?" "How do you stay motivated?" "How can I start?" Your answers will come from a place of deep experience and understanding, not theory. The lifestyle you live is a testimony to what's possible.

Your transformation highlights a key principle: when you align your diet, lifestyle, and goals with your physiology — when you work with your body instead of against it — change is not only achievable but sustainable. Naturally, there will be moments of temptation or stress, holidays or celebrations, travel or busy periods. But you have a tool kit now. You know how to navigate menus, say "yes" or "no" gracefully, and bring food that supports you. You know how to find balance and stay anchored in your choices.

Your ability to adapt and respond gracefully to these situations comes from a deep understanding of how your body performs best. It comes from honoring your signals — your hunger, your energy, your recovery — and making choices in service of those signals. It comes from choosing health over momentary indulgence and understanding that you're not depriving yourself; you're honoring yourself.

This path isn't about perfection; it's about progress. There will be moments when you eat something off plan, when you find yourself strayed from your routines. But those deviations will become less dramatic and less frequent, and you will learn to view them without shame or guilt — as small detours on a much larger journey — and you will find your way back quickly. That ability to course-correct gracefully is a powerful indicator of maturity and permanent lifestyle change.

Sustainability also comes from community and education. Staying connected to a group of people who share your goals — whether online, through a fitness class, or a health-oriented group — can help you stay motivated and supported. Continuing to learn more about nutrition, physiology, cooking, and meal planning lets you fine-tune your lifestyle and find strategies that align with your preferences. The more you know, the more proficient you become, and the less effort it feels like.

Your future health is a canvas you're coloring with each meal, each movement, each decision. The rich, satisfying foods you eat, the routines you maintain, and the choices you make all add depth and texture to your story. The discipline you cultivated, the knowledge you gained, and the confidence you earned will carry you forward, letting you pursue whatever goals you wish — whether it's physical fitness, sustained energy, a clear mind, or a deep peace with your own body.

Your 30-Day transformation was just the beginning. The greatest chapters are yet to come, and you have all the tools you need to make them remarkable. Your ketogenic lifestyle is not a temporary fix; it's a permanent renewal — a powerful affirmation of health, discipline, and self-determination. Whatever lies ahead, you're ready. The future is yours to conquer.

CHAPTER 30 — SUMMARY, INSPIRATION, AND ACTION PLAN

As you close this remarkable chapter in your journey, it's worth pausing for a moment to reflect on just how far you've come. The path you chose wasn't the path of least resistance. It wasn't a comfortable, convenient diet filled with shortcuts and promises of overnight transformation. It was a purposeful, powerful way of living — a lifestyle that demanded discipline, patience, adaptability, and deep resolve. And you responded by honoring your goals, honoring your health, and honoring yourself. The progress you made in just 30 days is a testament not only to a well-structured diet, but to your ability to follow through, to stay true to your intentions, and to conquer temptation in service of something greater.

This final chapter is a rich summary of everything you've learned and a powerful send-off into the future you're shaping for yourself. The ketogenic diet isn't a temporary fix; it's a permanent tool — a key you can use again and again to unlock health, energy, confidence, and well-being.

Picture for a moment all the small choices you made day after day. The moment you chose a handful of almonds over potato chips. The meal you prepared in advance instead of dialing for delivery. The time you walked away from temptation at a holiday dinner, choosing instead a plate filled with rich, savory foods that supported your goals. Each of these choices seemed small in the moment — barely a blip on the radar — but together, they made all the difference. Small choices add up. Small choices become habits. And habits become a lifestyle.

Your discipline and perseverance opened the door to a lifelong journey of health. The discipline wasn't a form of punishment; it was a form of freedom — freedom from cravings, from energy crashes, from poor health. It was a path toward a future filled with vitality, confidence, and renewal. The perseverance you cultivated over these 30 days made you realize something profoundly empowering: you are in control of your health. Your choices directly affect your future.

This final summary underscores all the key points you mastered — the power of a ketogenic diet to shift your metabolism from a carbohydrate-dependent state into a proficient, flexible, and efficient state of fatty acid utilization. It highlights meal planning strategies that kept you on track when temptation struck and busy schedules demanded adaptability. It underscores lifestyle choices — from staying adequately hydrated and well-supplemented, to honoring rest and recovery — that supported and amplified your progress.

Your future health, happiness, and confidence are now in your hands. There is no hidden formula you're missing; there is no "quick fix" you have yet to discover. The path forward lies in honoring what you know. It lies in staying the course, trusting the process, and making choices that align with your goals. Your future isn't something you passively wait for; it's something you create with each meal you eat, each movement you make, each decision you face.

This chapter guides you in formulating a clear action plan for your next steps. Whether you wish to stay strict ketogenic or ease into a more flexible low carbohydrate lifestyle, you have the knowledge and power to do it. If you wish to combine your diet with physical activity — adding resistance training, jogging, or yoga — now is a perfect time to find a regimen that fits your preferences and goals. If you wish to fine-tune your meal plan, adding back small amounts of carbohydrate from whole, rich sources, you know how to do it without backsliding into your former lifestyle.

Your future is filled with energy, clarity, and confidence. The lifestyle you have chosen lets you avoid the yo-yo dieting and health struggles that many people suffer from their whole lives. Instead, you have a powerful tool to maintain health and wellness for years to come. Your transformation signals not a temporary fix but a permanent change — a renewal — of body and mind.

Whatever path you pursue from here, you have all the knowledge you need to move forward. The greatest transformation you made wasn't just physical; it was a transformation of your habits, your choices, and your view of what you're capable of. The discipline you cultivated, the patience you maintained, the adaptability you demonstrated — all these traits will serve you well in whatever health journey you embark upon next.

The best part is — you're just getting started. There is a whole future of health, happiness, and confidence waiting for you. The choices you make from this day forward will reflect the person you have become. The person who made it through these 30 days. The person who chose discipline over temptation, future health over momentary indulgences, and transformation over stagnation.

So celebrate this moment. Celebrate your achievements and appreciate all the lessons you've learned. The future is yours to shape. Your transformation is not an ending — it's a beginning. Carry forward the knowledge, discipline, and confidence you have cultivated. Trust yourself, trust the process, and know that you are more than enough. The greatest chapters of your health journey lie just ahead.

Your future is not a straight road; it will have twists, detours, and moments of temptation. There will be days when you doubt yourself, when you find it hard to stay motivated, when you question whether all this discipline is worth it. But it's in those moments — the moments when you want to revert back to your old habits — that you will discover the true depth of your transformation. Your ability to stay true to your goals under pressure is what hardens discipline into character. It's what transforms you from someone who starts something new with a rush of motivation and drops it when the first obstacles arise, into someone who sees it through, no matter what. That, more than anything else, is the greatest triumph you have achieved in these 30 days.

Your discipline is a tool you can use in all areas of your life. The patience you cultivated while letting your body adjust, the adaptability you demonstrated by swapping ingredients or choosing healthy options on a restaurant menu — all these skills translate far beyond diet. They empower you to pursue goals in your career, relationships, fitness, and education with the same resolve you applied here. There is a deep synergy between honoring your health and honoring all your potential in life.

Picture yourself a year from now. Where will you be if you stay true to this path? Your energy will be sustained and strong. Your physical health will reflect your choices; you will move with ease, free from many of the ailments and discomforts you may have previously dealt with. Your confidence will permeate all you do, a quiet, powerful confidence born from having kept a promise to yourself. That confidence will affect your relationships, your ability to pursue goals, and your willingness to say "yes" to opportunities you previously may have avoided. Your discipline will become a powerful thread tying together all your future successes.

As you move forward, remember the strategies you mastered during this journey. Lean into meal planning and prepping; keep a well-stocked refrigerator and a clear meal calendar. Be kind but firm with yourself when temptation strikes — it's not a moral failing to be tempted, it's human — but choosing health over temptation is a powerful affirmation of your goals.

Support and community will remain key components of your future success. Lean on your friends, family, or online groups who share your lifestyle. Celebrate their progress and allow their stories to inspire you. Support is not weakness; it's a recognition that we are all interconnected and we grow stronger together.

As you find your stride in this lifestyle, consider mentoring someone else. Your experience — your struggles, your solutions, your triumphs — can become a powerful guide for a friend or family member who wants to pursue health but doesn't know where to start. Giving back in this way not only solidifies your own knowledge and discipline; it also lets you become a leader, a role model, a person who sparks transformation in others.

Your future health is a legacy you're building — not just for yourself, but for future generations. The choices you make today affect not only your own well-being but also the health patterns and attitudes your children, your family, and your community will carry forward. By honoring your health, you create a ripple of transformation that extends far beyond your own plate.

This lifestyle, this way of honoring your body and honoring yourself, is a powerful form of resistance against a world that often values instant satisfaction over sustained well-being. It's a vote for your future, for a life lived fully, without the limits that poor health can impose.

Your discipline will be tested, again and again. There will be holidays filled with rich food, social events where temptation is all around you, stressors that undermine your resolve. But you have something now that you did not have 30 days ago — you have knowledge, discipline, a deep understanding of your body's signals, and a powerful "why" to anchor you when temptation pulls you off course.

Your "why"—your deep, powerful reasons for choosing health over indulgence—should be something you reflect on frequently. Write it down and put it somewhere you will see it daily. Whenever temptation calls, return to your "why"—your children, your future, your happiness, your ability to pursue your passions without physical limitations. That "why" will cut through temptation and reconnect you with your goals.

Your plateaus, your struggles, your doubts — all these will come again, and that's okay. The key is not avoiding them but meeting them with a powerful, well-prepared mind. If you find you're stalling, reassess your diet. Are hidden carbohydrates creeping back in? Are you consuming more calories than you realize? Are you managing stress, honoring rest, staying adequately hydrated, and honoring all the components of health we discussed?

Your ability to navigate these obstacles gracefully will determine whether you revert back to old habits or break through into a new future. Each trial is an opportunity to grow, to learn, and to become more proficient at this lifestyle. Over time, staying ketogenic, honoring your health, and choosing discipline will become less effort and more habit — a rich, automatic way of living.

Ultimately, this journey isn't about punishment or shame; it's about honoring your body, honoring your future, and honoring yourself. It's a powerful form of self-love — choosing foods, habits, and routines that reflect your highest values.

Your future will be filled with rich experiences made possible by this discipline. Hiking a trail without getting winded, playing with children or grandchildren without tiring, traveling without health anxieties, wearing clothes you feel comfortable and proud in — all these things become a reality when you stay true to this path.

Your transformation is not a temporary diet; it's a permanent change in how you nourish yourself, physically and mentally. The chapters you have lived through in these 30 days are the foundation for many more chapters filled with health, happiness, and fulfillment.

So move forward with confidence, discipline, patience, and a deep understanding of what you're truly capable of. The future is yours to create — meal by meal, choice by choice, day by day — and there's no limit to what you can become.

www.ingramcontent.com/pod-product-compliance
Lightning Source LLC
La Vergne TN
LVHW090354210926
848480LV00002B/340